Intermittent Fasting
and
Ketogenic Diet

*How to Use Fasting to Optimize
Your Ketogenic Diet: Get Leaner,
Stronger, Healthier, and Better
Results in Less Time*

Nick Jackson

Table of Contents

Furthermore, the transmission, duplication or reproduction of any of the following work including specific information will be considered an illegal act irrespective of if it is done electronically or in print. This extends to creating a secondary or tertiary copy of the work or a recorded copy and is only allowed with the express written consent of the Publisher. All additional right reserved.

The information in the following pages is broadly considered to be a truthful and accurate account of facts and as such any inattention, use or misuse of the information in question by the reader will render any resulting actions solely under their purview. There are no scenarios in which the publisher or the original author of this work can be in any fashion deemed liable for any hardship or damages that may befall them after undertaking information described herein.

Additionally, the information in the following pages is intended only for informational purposes and should thus be thought of as universal. As befitting its nature, it is presented without assurance regarding its prolonged validity or interim quality. Trademarks that are mentioned are done without written consent and can in no way be considered an endorsement from the trademark holder.

Introduction

Congratulations on downloading this book and thank you for doing so. You're already on you're way to being much more badass than you already are. By following the protocols listed in this book, you will dramatically increase your HGH, optimize your hormones (testosterone if you're a man), reduce body fat, think more clearly, have clearer skin, and feel like a complete badass. It's true!!!! The dieting methods described in this book will have you feeling like a superhero and you'll reap more health benefits than you ever thought possible (without a magic pill anyway). So, let's getting started showing you how to be unleash your inner badass with some simple dietary modifications.

The following chapters will discuss exactly what is entailed in a ketogenic diet and more importantly, how to incorporate intermittent fasting with a ketogenic diet to dramatically augment your fat burning and muscle building capabilities. You will also learn what makes ketogenic dieting and intermittent fasting work. You will learn the basic mechanisms behind how the body works when it must operate on low-carbohydrates and when it operates in a fasted state. You will also learn how incorporating these strategies will help you to burn more fat and effectively build more muscle mass.

There will be a chapter covering the many benefits to be gained from converting over to a ketogenic diet. You will learn how this type of diet can help lower blood pressure, increase your energy throughout the day, think more clearly, and how it aids in effectively and efficiently burning fat while maintaining your muscle mass.

There will be also be a chapter covering the many benefits of intermittent fasting. You will learn how intermittent fasting increases human growth hormone (HGH), how it protects your brain and enables more mental clarity, how it allows you to naturally detox your body, and how it may just be the fountain of youth. The many benefits of intermittent fasting are just now being realized and its promise is great.

As well, you will learn how to implement ketogenic dieting along with intermittent fasting to optimize your results. You will soon have a dieting combination that works to burn more fat, build

more muscle, and provides more benefits than either strategy alone. By utilizing these two highly effective strategies,
you'll be able to get faster and better results. I'll teach you the best ways to use
these strategies together. I'll even show
you how you can use these two strategies
to have a successful cheat day without
sacrificing all your hard work. By the
time you finish this book, you'll be able
to eat better, look better, feel better, and
be better.

Chapter 1: What Is The Ketogenic Diet?

The ketogenic or keto diet is synonymous with a low carb diet. Although, it is true that all ketogenic diets are low carb in nature, not all low carbohydrate diets are ketogenic. There is, however, most definitely some overlap. This will be explained in greater detail later. However, for now, know that the ketogenic diet is by definition a diet that characterized by the production of ketones.

As stated previously, the ketogenic diet works by forcing the body to produce ketones. It does this through a metabolic state known as ketosis, which is a naturally occurring physiological state that controls and regulates ketone bodies produced within the body. This is a totally harmless physiological state when it is used properly in a ketogenic diet. In fact as you'll learn, it's really quite beneficial. Dietary ketosis is what gets your body to use ketone bodies as fuel as opposed to using carbohydrates. Burning ketone bodies and fatty acids is one of the most efficient ways the body can use energy. Ketosis works by producing fuel from fat and thus decreasing the amount of fat in your body.

The ketogenic diet creates a hormonal state in the body that is conducive to fat burning and detoxification. By restricting carbohydrates and forcing the body to deplete its sugar reserves, the body enters ketosis and a state of repair known as autophagy. This state of autophagy is also seen with fasting and is one of the shared benefits of these two dietary strategies. Autophagy is basically a cleaning state in which the body consumes its dying and damaged cells. This results in a fat burning diet that not only allows you to get the body you want on the outside but on the inside as well. By using this diet, you will detoxify your body, optimize your hormone levels, reduce inflammation, enhance brain function, and increase energy levels. A lot of these benefits come from the ketogenic nature of the diet and that makes this diet unique and better than alternatives. In fact, the ketogenic diet isn't a diet for its proponents; it's a way of life.

Chapter 2: How Does Keto Dieting Work?

The ketogenic diet works because it is scientifically sound and it exploits the mechanisms how the body converts food into fuel for energy. To understand how the keto diet works, you first must understand what a carbohydrate is and what it does in the body.

What are Carbohydrates?

Carbohydrates are macronutrients that are found in a wide variety of foods. What is a macronutrient? Macronutrients are basically nutrients in substantial quantities that the body needs. There are three macronutrients; carbohydrates, fats, and proteins. The calories that you consume from macronutrients are what generates energy in the body. Carbohydrates are an excellent source of fuel for the brain and help to preserve ingested protein so that it can be converted into muscle mass.

Carbohydrates can be a powerhouse energy source for the body. Therefore, it is important to understand which carbohydrates are best for consumption because some carbohydrates are better for you than others. This is especially true if you plan on utilizing carbohydrates as fuel for energy. Carbohydrates can be found in numerous processed foods. The carbohydrates in these foods are typically simple sugars, which tend to be the carbohydrates that you should try to stay away from.

Plant-based foods usually have naturally occurring carbohydrates. These are the carbohydrates that you want to be consuming. These will be your vegetables, fruits, legumes, seeds, and nuts. The goal here will be to choose the best variety of these options to consume; which we will go over in a later chapter.

Types of Carbohydrates

There are three main categories of carbohydrates; fiber, sugar, and starches. Simple carbohydrates or sugars are the simplest forms of carbohydrates. Many foods have naturally occurring sugars; milk sugar which is known as lactose, fructose which is fruit sugar, and sucrose which is generally referred to as table sugar.

Complex carbohydrates or starches are naturally occurring in foods like grains, beans, and vegetables. The difference between simple and complex carbohydrates is the way that they are structured chemically. Complex carbohydrates contain numerous sugar molecules bonded together. You can think of this as many sugar molecules linked together in a chain. Note that the types of carbohydrates that you want to consume should be the minimally or unprocessed versions of these foods. Complex carbohydrates are going to give you an extended amount of energy and help you increase your glycogen storages.

Fiber is a type of complex carbohydrate that can also be found naturally in foods. Fiber is an exception to the way that complex carbohydrates work since the body is unable to digest this type of carbohydrate. Although dietary fiber is not digested and broken down for energy, it is very beneficial to your health. Fiber can either be soluble or insoluble. Insoluble fibers do not dissolve in water while soluble fibers will dissolve in water. These specific characteristics of fiber allow it to greatly benefit the body. For instance, soluble fiber tends to bind to and decrease cholesterol levels while insoluble fiber bulks stool. Altogether, fiber helps to aid in digestion (by keeping you regular), helps regulate cholesterol and blood sugar levels, and suppresses appetite.

What Exactly is Ketosis?

Now that you have a general understanding of what a carbohydrate is and how it works, you can now start to apply the principles of ketogenic dieting. Keto dieting will allow your body to efficiently utilize fat as your primary energy source. This occurs by limiting your carbohydrate intake and allowing your body to burn up all of its glycogen stores.

When carbohydrates are consumed, they are broken down into glucose for immediate energy needs. The body will then secrete insulin which enables the body to process the glucose. If fat is consumed with the carbohydrates, it is stored since the glucose is used for immediate energy needs. Any excess glucose is stored as well, in the form of glycogen.

Glycogen is the storage form of glucose and is present in the muscles and in the liver. Think as of glycogen as your fuel tank, in the absence of glucose, the body will use its glycogen stores for immediate energy needs. As well, during high intensity exercise, your muscle glycogen stores are preferentially burned up to fuel your muscles. When you body has exhausted all of its glycogen stores, it must start tapping into its fat stores to meet its energy demands. When the body starts burning its fat, it goes into ketosis. Ketosis is a physiological process in which ketones are produced by the body. Ketones, or ketone bodies, are the byproducts of fat breakdown and are a preferential fuel source for the brain and nervous tissue.

Ketones

Ketones, or ketone bodies, are the byproducts of fatty acids that are metabolized in the liver. Why is the production of ketones so important and why should I care? Well the answer to this intriguing question is answered in the paragraph below.

Once the body realizes carbohydrate sources are limited, it begins to break down its glycogen stores to produce energy for the body. When glycogen sources are depleted it begins to enter the state of ketosis where it begins to breakdown adipose tissue, otherwise known as fat, in order to produce energy for the body. While the fatty acids that are released from fat are able to provide fuel for most of the body, it is unable to produce the glucose that the brain requires for energy. Without carbohydrates available to provide the glucose the brain needs, the body will resort to breaking down its protein (which can be metabolized to glucose) to meet these needs. Therefore, muscle mass (your body's most readily available protein storage) can and will be broken down to form the glucose the brain needs. This is not a good thing, unless you want your muscle mass to waste away, your metabolism to plummet, and your strength to decrease as you lose weight. However, ketone bodies, which are produced from the fatty acids that are liberated from adipose tissue or through ingested fat, can act like an energy source for the brain as well.

The overall goal of this diet is to be able to use fat as energy. By keeping our glycogen levels depleted and our carbohydrate intakes low, we will stay in ketosis and reap the benefits of a ketogenic diet. By eating a high fat diet, we will keep our energy levels up and allow our bodies to get very efficient at burning fat. This whole process of becoming efficient at burning fat and switching from a carbohydrate burning metabolism to a fat burning metabolism is know in the keto and low carbohydrate world as becoming fat adapted.

Chapter 3: Benefits of the Ketogenic Diet

There are many benefits to be gained from using a ketogenic diet that can be helpful to a variety of individuals. From world class athletes to individuals with medical conditions, a ketogenic diet has been proven to have numerous beneficial values. As with any diet, especially if you have any medical conditions, you should first consult with your doctor to confirm whether this type of diet is right for you. For the majority of individuals, implementing a ketogenic diet will most likely lead to an overall more balanced and healthier lifestyle.

Weight Loss

Arguably the best and most attractive benefit for adhering to a ketogenic diet. Compared to other diets, using a ketogenic diet will help you lose more weight.   First off, when you first start limiting your carbohydrate intake, you will burn through your glycogen stores and this will result in a dramatic weight loss. This is the water weight that most people lose when first starting low carbohydrate diets. This occurs since each gram of glycogen that is burned causes the body to release 3 grams of water (since 3 grams of water are attached to each gram of glycogen). This results in a rapid loss of water weight that may be anywhere from 5 to 15 pounds for most people. This loss of water weight is part of the reason why people look leaner on low carb diets and is why people lose so much weight in the first week.   However, once the body becomes fat adapted and begin to utilize fat and ketones as its main fuel sources, it will be a fat burning machine. The faster you can get the body into ketosis, the faster you will be able to burn more fat resulting in an overall loss of body weight. The great benefit to this is that since the body is relying on ketones and fat for energy all the weight loss will be fat loss, helping you to retain and minimize muscle loss.

Another great benefit to ketogenic dieting is that it is easy to stay on. By eating more fat and protein than the typical diets, you will not be hungry even when in a caloric deficit. It has been proven that high protein and high fat diets are more filling than low fat diets. Ultimately, this diet is the most effective you can undertake and definitely the easiest to stick to.

How do ketogenic diets compare to other diets?

It is important to know that the production of ketones and the body's process of becoming "fat adapted" is paramount to the success of ketogenic diets. In fact, this sets it apart from diets that are not ketogenic in nature. This is because diets that are higher in carbohydrates will burn up muscle protein to produce glucose for the brain once immediate energy stores are exhausted. While proponents of higher carbohydrate diets will say that the inclusion of significant and constant carbohydrate sources will minimize this; in the presence of a calorie deficit, you will tap into your protein stores at sometime. The ketogenic diet minimizes this process as the body goes through enzymatic changes during ketosis that makes the body more efficient at burning fat. Your fat and the fat that you eat become the primary energy sources in ketosis. These fatty acids are metabolized into ketones, which supply the brain with the energy it needs. Therefore, ketosis spares your muscle protein while burning fat.

Muscle Gain

The wonderful thing about implementing a ketogenic diet is the fact that while you lose weight, you can also begin to increase your muscle mass. This is especially enticing to athletes, bodybuilders, and anyone who wants to increase or pack on muscle. By implementing a ketogenic diet along with an exercise regimen, it becomes easy to build muscle mass. This is especially true for men on a ketogenic diet since high fat diets will cause a natural increase in testosterone. Therefore, an appropriately designed ketogenic diet will have men burning through their fat stores while using their protein intake to build muscle.

Increased Energy and More Satiety

Since your body will be tapping into its fat stores and using ingested fat for energy, it will have a more consistent and reliable energy source. Everyone has experienced the tiredness and fatigue that a meal rich in carbohydrates can produce. This is because of blood sugar fluctuations due to the secretion of insulin. Without the influence of carbohydrates on your blood sugar, you will find that you have a steady source of energy and less fatigue throughout the day.

Blood Pressure and Cholesterol

Ketogenic diets have been proven to help lower cholesterol levels and blood pressure. This is particularly helpful with individuals that have built up plaque in their arteries due to abnormal triglyceride levels and cholesterol levels. With individuals who have high blood pressure related to an excess of weight, a ketogenic diet may contribute to weight loss which will cause a decrease in blood pressure. As well, ketogenic diets tend to be dehydrating and people will not retain as much fluid on a ketogenic diet. This leads to a reduction in blood pressure via reduced fluid retention. Therefore, this type of diet can be very beneficial to individuals who have medical conditions that directly affect blood pressure and cholesterol levels.

Controlling Diabetes

This disease is the result of the body becoming less responsive to the effects of insulin. This causes the body to be unable to process glucose and the clinical symptoms of diabetes is the result. One of the biggest risk factors for developing Diabetes Mellitus Type II is being overweight. For these individuals converting over to a ketogenic diet, it not only assists with weight loss but it will also help lower insulin levels. The purpose of the ketogenic diet is for the body to use fat as an energy source not carbohydrates or glucose. By implementing this diet and changing your lifestyle, the body will naturally reduce the need for insulin which can help maintain a steady, normal level of glucose in the blood. Low carb diets in general have been shown to increase insulin sensitivity and can be used in early diabetics to reverse or at least control their diabetes.

Improving Mental Focus

Improved mental focus and concentration is a known result of ketogenic dieting. This occurs because the brain and nervous system usually relies upon glucose to meet their energy needs. However, this changes when carbohydrate levels begin to get low and the liver begins to produce ketone bodies. When this occurs, ketone bodies become the primary source of fuel for the brain. With the brain having a steady flow of ketone bodies for energy, you can use that reliable source of energy to help assist you with effectively concentrating and focusing on tasks. This is a great benefit as a carb laden diet can cause blood sugar spikes and crashes, which can affect focus and energy levels. With a ketogenic diet, this is never a problem as blood sugar is more tightly regulated and blood sugar stays within a tight range. For these reasons, many individuals incorporate a ketogenic diet to help improve their mental performance.

Conditions, Diseases, and Disorders

Ketogenic diets have successfully been shown to help minimize the symptoms of some medical illnesses; diabetes and high blood pressure are just a couple that have already been discussed. As well, ketogenic diets are being investigated as potential therapies for a wide range of neurological disorders. Right now, there is mounting evidence that ketogenic diets, particularly the metabolic shift that results in ketone bodies being the preferred energy source for the brain, can exert neuroprotective activity within the brain. Some animal and cell studies have shown that ketone bodies may exert antioxidant properties, which lead to a healthier mind. In fact, ketogenic diets have been shown to be useful in epilepsy and are an effective treatment for people with medically refractory epilepsy. Currently, it is hypothesized and being investigated as a possible treatment for neurological diseases and conditions such as migraine, Parkinson Disease, Alzheimer Disease, ALS, brain trauma, and many more. While more studies are needed to confirm the utility of ketogenic diets for many of these conditions, the ability of this diet to affect brain energy metabolism makes it very promising for future therapies.

Acne

One benefit that can be observed fairly quickly while ketogenic dieting is a better complexion. People tend to find that once they get on a ketogenic diet, they will see less facial blemishes and acne. In fact, zits and acne are a thing of the past on this lifestyle. This can be explained by the studies linking high carbohydrate intake to acne. As well, low carbohydrate diets have been shown to decrease skin inflammation. By following a ketogenic diet, people can minimize the potential triggers from foods that may be contributing to acne. This is a great and immediate benefit for many people who struggle with facial blemishes, acne, and facial break outs. These people can expect to see the results from the ketogenic diet soon after adopting it just by looking in the mirror.

Chapter 4: Common Ketogenic Diet Side Effects

Now that we know that the keto diet is all that and a bag of chips (well maybe not exactly a bag of chips!!), we need to talk about the possible unpleasantries that may be associated with starting a keto diet. Don't worry, for the most part these are temporary and can easily be combatted. These issues and how to deal with them are listed below.

Keto Flu

This common side effect occurs when you are first starting out on a ketogenic diet. You may experience fatigue, nausea, cramps, aching, poor concentration, head ache, and overall like you've come down with something. These symptoms have come to be referred to as the keto flu. This is transient and will only last 4 to 5 days while your body is getting accustomed to ketosis. During this time, you are likely to feel drained but once your body transitions over to a fat adapted ketogenic state you will have more energy than ever.

Just because the keto flu is common doesn't mean there aren't ways to eliminate it or reduce the severity of this condition. A lot of these symptoms are from dehydration and lost electrolytes as your body is losing a lot of water weight through its depletion of glycogen. This tends to leave people deficient in magnesium, potassium, and sodium. By drinking a powerade zero or other sugar free electrolyte enriched drink, you can stop a lot of these symptoms. Make sure you are taking a multivitamin and mineral supplement and increase your fluid intake. Just by doing this, you will likely prevent the keto flu.

Constipation

This is a big one for many people undergoing a ketogenic diet. By restricting carbohydrates, people tend to cut out a lot of their sources of fiber. This along with an increased chance of dehydration will lead to constipation. This is easily combated by increasing your fluid intake and ensuring that you are eating plenty of low carb fibrous veggies. If you want to skip the veggies, ensure you are taking a sugar free fiber supplement. Personally, I like to go with benefiber as it is essentially tasteless and mixes well with any liquid. Make sure you are also taking a greens supplement if you are not eating enough veggies so that you don't miss out on all of the benefits of this food group.

Cramps

Many people experience muscle cramps when on a ketogenic diet. These will generally occur early in the morning or late at night and during exercise. This occurs due to electrolyte and fluid depletion. Once again, to prevent this side effect, just ensure you are replenishing your electrolytes and drinking plenty of fluids. Due to the dehydrating tendencies of this diet, I highly advise propel or powerade zero consumption during any workout.

Poor Physical Performance

Another common side effect of initiating a ketogenic diet is poor physical performance. When you first start the keto diet, expect to be more tired and to have fatigue. Working out will seem like a chore and when you do it, you will feel weak and tire easily. However, this is short-lived. The great news is that this piss poor performance and tiredness is replaced almost over night with more energy and more endurance. Once your body gets used to running on fat for energy, you will have less energy lulls and you'll be more energetic. Your strength will come back and you'll notice that your performance will be better than ever. It may take a week or two to be completely fat adapted and running one hundred percent on your fat reserves but it's definitely worth it.

Ketone Breath

When you are in ketosis, you body will secrete ketones through your breath and other bodily fluids. You will definitely notice this when you are in ketosis. Your urine will be highly pungent.

Marking your territory would be no problem when you are in this metabolic state because your piss will smell horrible. As well, you will often have a sweet taste in your mouth as you excrete the ketone acetone through your breath. This will also give your breath a distinct odor. This side effect of ketone breath can be masked by chewing sugar-free gum.

Ketoacidosis

It is important to note that there is a serious medical condition known as ketoacidosis. This medical condition can be fatal and is characterized by excess and unregulated ketones in the bloodstream. For most people, who are healthy, this is not a concern. The is because the body closely regulates its fat metabolism and will rarely produce more ketones than it needs to function.

Your body is designed to metabolize and process these ketone bodies. However, this can be a concern with uncontrolled diabetics, who have elevated blood sugar, or in people with acute alcohol intoxication and underlying disorders. It should be noted that even diabetics can use low carb dieting to control their blood sugar and decrease the need for medications, but it is advised that they do so only under close medical supervision.

Chapter 5: Implementing the Ketogenic Diet

When you make the decision to undertake a ketogenic diet, there are ways that you can help yourself incorporate new foods as well as eliminate the foods that essentially have no nutritional value. The first thing you should do is determine the amount of carbohydrates, protein, and fat that you need to consume each day. This can be done with some easy to follow guidelines.

Calorie Requirements

The first thing to do in setting up your ketogenic diet is to figure up how many calories you need to be eating daily. This is going to be dependent upon whether you want to lose weight, maintain, or gain weight. There are a couple of ways of figuring out how many calories you should be eating daily and most of these will use your lean body mass. However, we can get a fairly accurate estimation by multiplying your bodyweight by a corresponding multiplier based on activity level. We can then adjust our measurements and food intake based on our results.

To determine the amount of calories we should shoot for daily, multiply your bodyweight in pounds by one of the following multipliers based on activity level; 12-14 for sedentary individuals, 14-16 for moderately active (3-4 times weekly exercise), and 16-18 for very active (5-7 times weekly exercise). These values will give you the amount of calories you need to take in daily just to maintain your weight. This number, know as your maintenance level of calories, can then be adjusted to meet your goals. Since there are 3500 calories in a pound of fat, we can subtract 500 calories daily from our maintenance level of calories for each pound of fat we'd like to lose weekly (3500 calories/7 days= 500 calories/day). So, in order to lose 2 pound a week, one would just need to subtract 1000 calories from their daily maintenance level of calories.

For example, a 200 pound person that doesn't workout or have a very physical job would need to consume between 2400 to 2800 calories (200 lbs X 12 calories/lb = 2400 calories and 200 lbs X 14 calories/lb = 2800 calories) daily to maintain weight on a ketogenic diet. In order to lose 2 pounds of weight weekly, this person would start by taking in 1800 calories weekly and then adjust their calories based on their results.

If someone wanted to gain muscle mass on a ketogenic diet, it is advised to eat 250-500 calories daily over their maintenance level of calories in order to gain muscle mass while minimizing fat gain. So, our 200 pound individual who is now moderately active and lifting weights to gain muscle mass would need to be taking in 3450 calories daily (200 lbs X 16 calories/lb =3200 calories, 3200 calories + 250 calories = 3450 calories).

With all of these estimations of calories, it is prudent to keep careful track of your calories daily so you may ascertain what is happening if you are not getting the results you want. For instance, if you estimated you need to be eating 2000 calories daily to lose 2 pounds a week but you are not losing any then you'd have a way to examine your caloric intake. You will need to ensure you calorie measurements are accurate then adjust from there. You may need to add or subtract calories based on your weekly progress and your goals. Be sure that you are not hasty though. I advise cutting calories further only after 2 weeks of stalled progress and after you have added in additional activity. As well, when you are working on gaining muscle mass, start low and go slow so that you don't pack on additional fat.

Body Fat Percentage

The next thing to do when setting up your ketogenic diet is to determine your body fat percentage. This is imperative to determining your protein intake. The added benefit of being able to track your results also makes this an essential thing to do. I go into great detail about determining body fat percentage in my first book <u>Rapid Fat Loss Mastery: Lose Weight While Retaining Muscle at an Incredible Rate</u>. This is also a great diet to jump start a keto diet or get fast results. I just had to put that shameless plug in there. Anyhow, the quick and dirty method the I recommend to determine your body fat percentage is using a one-site accu-measure body fat caliper. This is easy to use and can be found online for approximately ten dollars. Other methods, such as the YMCA method and the US Navy method will give you a ball park estimate of body fat percentage based on your height, weight, gender, and waist measurements. These calculators can be found easily online with a google search.

Lean Body Mass

Once you've determined your body fat percentage, you will use this number to determine your lean body mass. Your lean body mass or lbm is a measure of the amount of lean tissue on your body. This measurement is essentially all the tissues on your body minus your fat stores. Thus, you can figure out this number by subtracting your fat weight from your total body weight. So, multiply your body fat percentage by your body weight to determine the amount of fat you are carrying and then subtract this number from your total body weight to get your lean body mass. So, if a 200 pound person finds that they 10% body fat, they will have 20 pounds of fat and 180 pounds of lean body mass. The calculation for pounds of fat with this example is as follows: 200 lbs X .10= 20 lbs fat. To calculate lean body mass, this number is just subtracted from total body weight: 200 lbs - 20 lbs = 180 lbs.

LBM: Total Body weight - (Total Body Weight X Body Fat %)

Protein Requirements

The first macronutrient that needs to be calculated is your protein requirement. This number will vary depending up your personal goals and workout strategy. It is absolutely essential to get enough protein to prevent muscle break down and to meet the demands of the body. However, too much protein can inhibit ketosis as protein can be converted to glucose via gluconeogenesis. Therefore, in order to optimize our results, the following guidelines should be used: sedentary individuals should get between 0.6 to 0.8 grams of protein per pound of lean body mass, active individuals should aim for 0.8 to 1 gram of protein per pound of lbm, while people working out should get 1 to 1.2 grams per pound of lbm. Many people that are actively weight training will ensure they get 1 gram of protein per pound of body weight. As long as you are not significantly overweight, this shouldn't be enough protein to completely inhibit ketosis. However, if you are quite a bit overweight, it would be prudent to eat grams of protein closer to your lean body mass measurements.

I highly recommend determining your body fat percentage and knowing your exact protein requirement but I'm sure most people will not take the time to calculate their body fat percentage. So, to get an estimate of the amount of protein needed, we can assume an average body fat percentage and calculate our body fat based on these numbers. Obviously this number varies depending upon your age, sex, and workout history but we can assume an average body fat percentage of 25% for men and 30% for women. Using our 200 pound male example, our body fat percentage of 25% would give us 50 pounds of body fat (0.25 X 200 pounds = 50 pounds). Our lean body mass is calculated by subtracting our body fat from our weight. So, this individual would have 150 pounds of lean body mass. His protein requirement would be then be based off this number and his activity level. Assuming he decides to eat 1 gram per pound of lbm, he would aim to take in 150 grams of protein daily. Protein also has 4 calories per gram, therefore, he would need 600 calories daily in protein (4 calories per gram X 150 grams of protein = 600 calories of protein).

Carbohydrate Requirements

Now that we have determined how much protein to consume, we will determine how many carbohydrates to eat daily. We will attempt to keep our carbohydrate intake below 30 grams daily. Staying below this amount will ensure that we enter ketosis. The lower we keep our carbohydrates, the quicker and easier it will be to enter ketosis and begin burning up fat. When counting your grams of carbohydrates, you may subtract the grams of fiber from you carbohydrate counts. This is because fiber is included in the carbohydrate counts of foods but it is not absorbed by the body and will not affect your blood sugar or disrupt ketosis. For instance, if a protein bar label states that it contains 24 grams of carbohydrates and 14 grams of fiber, you would only count 10 grams of carbohydrates toward your daily total. You will also need to determine the amount of calories you are consuming from the total number of carbohydrate (fiber included here). There is a total of 4 calories per gram of carbohydrates. Therefore, you can determine how many calories you are taking in from carbohydrates by multiplying the number of carbs in grams by 4 calories. So, in general, you should be ingesting 120 calories or less of carbohydrates daily (4 calories/g carbs X 30 g carbs = 120 calories).

As mentioned previously, the ketogenic diet is a high fat, low carb, and moderate to high protein diet. On a typical ketogenic diet, it is generally recommended that your macronutrient intake come from 70-75% fats, 20-25% protein, and 5-10% carbohydrates. Of course, these percentages will vary depending upon your goals and personal preferences.

Fat Requirements

To figure out how much fat you need on the low carb portion of this diet, you would simply determine how many total calories you need daily and then ascertain how many grams of fat you need to meet your caloric requirements. For example, our 200 pound sedentary male needs 2400 calories daily. Assuming he's 25% body fat, he'd have 150 pounds of lbm. If we calculated his protein requirements using his activity level, he would need between 90-120 grams of protein daily (0.6 g X 150 g/lb = 90 g, 0.8 g X 150g/lb = 120 g). He is going to be getting 120 calories from carbs (using our 30 gram maximum) and up to 480 calories from protein (4 cal/g X 120 g = 480 calories). Therefore, he needs 1800 calories from fat to reach his daily requirement for calories (2400 daily calories - 600 carb & protein calories= 1800 calories). Since there is 9 calories for every gram of fat, he needs a total of 200 grams of fat daily (1800 calories/9 fat calories per gram = 200 grams of fat).

Alternative Macronutrient Planning Option

Finding your grams of macronutrients and planning your diet is crucial to your long term success on this diet, especially if you're using it to lose weight. However, if you decide this is too much effort, you can still get great results by monitoring your minimal daily protein intake while restricting your carbohydrates to less than 30 grams daily. By doing this and just eating until you are satisfied, you will likely still be eating in a calorie deficit and getting results. However, by not monitoring your calories daily, you will eventually plateau as your consumption approaches your maintenance level of calories. In order to make further progress, you will need to ensure you are eating less calories than you are expending. Even if you are monitoring your calories sufficiently, you will likely reach a point where you will plateau with weight loss. This is because as you lose weight, your body becomes more efficient at using calories and you need less calories overall. If you are using the diet for weight loss and you do not see results for 2 weeks in a row, decrease your total weekly calorie intake by 500 calories and proceed. The scale should start moving again with this approach.

Chapter 6: What to Eat

It is important to stick to your ketogenic diet consistently without deviation for the first couple of weeks. This will ensure that you become fat adapted and you get the best results. Some people may want to take a cheat meal or cheat day for psychological reasons or to build muscle. These strategies will be discussed later in the intermittent fasting portion of the book. The food choices that you should be making when in ketosis, however, are described below.

As explained earlier, your ketogenic diet will be one that is high in fat, moderate to high in protein, and extremely low in carbohydrates. Therefore, your diet will be predominantly composed of high fat protein sources, fatty dressings, and low carbohydrate veggies. There will be absolutely no refined or processed sugars at all and likely no room for fruits either.

Fruits and Vegetables

Due to the sugar content of fruits, it is advisable to not eat any. As well, it is very important to choose your vegetables wisely when on a ketogenic diet. You want to choose the vegetables that are low in carbohydrates but are also high in nutrients. These are typically going to be your large green leafy vegetables.

A quick note about vegetables to help you decide whether it is an appropriate choice for your diet, a good rule of thumb is to consider if the vegetable tastes sweet or not. Typically, the sweeter a vegetable tastes, the more sugar the vegetable has in it. These would be the vegetables you want to stay away from as they would have a higher carbohydrate content. Remember to check labels and carbohydrate content of any and all veggies you want to incorporate into your diet. You should strive to get less than 30 grams of net carbohydrates throughout the day. Green leafy veggies are generally high in fiber and low in carbohydrates and should therefore be your primary sources.

Here is a list of commonly used vegetables that you should consider incorporating into your diet.

- asparagus
- bell pepper
- broccoli
- brussels sprouts
- cabbage
- cucumber
- cauliflower
- mushrooms

- onions
- celery
- radish
- kale
- s w i s s
- m i x e d
  chard
  greens
- tomatoes
- okra

Protein

You should be consuming an adequate amount of protein every day with your ketogenic diet. This is especially important because the intake of protein helps assist with the building up of muscle mass. Proteins should make up the largest portion of your meals. Animal meats, fish, eggs, and high fat dairy should be the bulk of your menu here. These foods will be satiating and will allow you to attain your fat requirements for the day as well. Vegetarians and vegans can also adopt a ketogenic diet. The protein you consume does not need to come from animals as there are many alternatives to animal products.

Here is a list of commonly used protein rich foods:

- beef
- dairy
- fish
- goat
- lamb
- offal (organ meat)
- pork
- poultry
- shellfish
- tofu
- turkey
- veal
- whole eggs

When choosing which cut of meat to use, ensure you are picking a fattier selection. Hamburger, steak, beef, and bacon are all great options. If you opt for chicken, make sure you fry it up in lard and keep that delicious skin on it.

When selecting a type of fish, you should aim for ones that are captured in the wild. Fresh fish is ideal so if there is a market where you can purchase fresh fish, try to purchase those options over the frozen fish options. Common fish used in ketogenic diets include sardines, salmon, mackerel, catfish, snapper, cod, mahi-mahi, trout, and tuna.

For some vegetarians, nut butter and eggs can be a reliable source of protein. When it comes to using eggs as protein, the whole egg should be used. If possible, try to get free range eggs if available. Eggs are one of the most versatile foods because they can be cooked several different ways. As well, eggs have a good deal of fat and are a great protein source. Definitely use eggs to your advantage. For vegans, nut butter and egg substitutes can be used for protein. If you choose to incorporate nut butter, choose the unsweetened and natural varieties.

Legumes, Nuts, and Seeds

Use caution when choosing to add nuts to your meals since their carbohydrate content can add up quickly. Nuts are high in fat and protein which you should also consider when developing your meal plans.

Here is a list of commonly used legumes, nuts, and seeds for ketogenic diets:

- almonds
- brazil nuts
- chia
- flaxseed
- hazelnuts
- macadamia nuts
- pecans

Nuts that you could consume in moderation include almonds, pine nuts, walnuts, and peanuts. Since the ketogenic diet calls for no processed foods, flour is not an option. There are many alternatives to the white and wheat flours. Some of these include; coconut flour, chia seed meal, almond flour, and flaxseed meal. Flaxseed meal is also a great alternative to white flour and it also provides you with dietary fiber.

Dairy Products

Depending on how strict you are on your ketogenic diet, you may want to choose to incorporate dairy. Although there are low-fat and fat-free options when it comes to dairy products, always choose the full-fat products over the others. The full-fat dairy products generally have significantly lower amounts of carbohydrates compared to the low-fat and fat-free versions. Being rich with calcium, which has been shown to increase fat burning, these full-fat dairy products also typically tend to be more satiating.

Here is a list of commonly used dairy products consumed on a ketogenic diet:

- aged cheese
- blue cheese
- brie
- Colby cheese
- cottage cheese
- feta cheese
- grass-fed butter
- ghee
- Greek yogurt
- heavy whipping cream
- mascarpone
- mayonnaise
- mozzarella
- parmesan
- sour cream
- swiss cheese

There are many alternatives to dairy products for individuals who may have sensitivities to lactose. Coconut milk and almond milk can be great alternatives for these individuals. Some yogurts, kefir, goat's milk, and aged cheese are other options for individuals who have lactose sensitivities.

Beverages and Water

Water should be the number one thing that you drink every day, regardless of your diet. This is especially true when you are on a ketogenic diet. As humans, we are roughly made up of about 70% water which goes to show you how important it is to drink water.

Dehydration is very common among individuals who start a ketogenic diet because it naturally has a diuretic effect on the body. This happens because you deplete your glycogen stores due to the low carb phase of the diet. Each gram of glycogen contains 3 grams of water. Thus, as you lose your glycogen, your body loses water along with it. This leads to a substantial amount of water weight loss. As well, the increased protein that is taken in during a ketogenic diet results in a larger amount of urea being produced, which is a by-product of protein metabolism. This is flushed out of the body as urine. This basically means that a ketogenic diet will cause you to lose a lot of water weight, most likely in the form of urine production. For this reason, it is very important that you consume an adequate amount of water daily.

What is an adequate amount of daily water consumption? This should be around 8 glasses of 8 ounces of water for a total of at least 64 ounces of water a day. Remember that if you are thirsty, you are already dehydrated. So drink plenty of fluids daily. The best way to ensure you are staying hydrated is to monitor the color of your urine output. Your urine should be clear to straw colored in appearance. Any darker than this and you are showing signs of dehydration.

Here is a list of commonly consumed beverages for a ketogenic diet:

- almond milk
- broth
- diet soda
- coffee
- coconut milk
- soy milk
- tea

Coffee and tea are popular among individuals on ketogenic diets. If you do choose to incorporate coffee and tea into your ketogenic diet, go for black coffee and green tea whenever possible. If you want to use a creamer for your coffee or tea, make sure that you use low to no sugar creamers. Unsweetened almond or coconut milk are good options. Diet soda, as long as it is calorie-free, is also perfectly fine to drink on a ketogenic diet.

Fats and Oils

When you think about adding fats and oils to your meals, you want to make sure that you choose the healthier options for both. You want to choose naturally occurring polyunsaturated fats, saturated fats, and monounsaturated fats. The wrong types of fats can cause serious medical conditions and problems but consuming fats are a vital part of daily nutrition.

The Omega-3 fatty acids are excellent sources of essential fatty acids. These fatty acids are commonly found in shellfish and fish like tuna and salmon. If possible, try to incorporate these types of foods into your diet. When choosing what oils and fats to purchase, look for the grass-fed and organic varieties whenever available.

Here is a list of commonly used oils and fats on a ketogenic diet:

- avocado oil
- avocados
- butter
- cocoa butter
- coconut butter
- egg yolks
- lard
- olive oil

- palm oil
- macadamia oil
- MCT oil
- non-hydro-genated an-imal fat

When using oils, you should choose the cold pressed options whenever possible. These include canola, olive, sesame, coconut, and sunflower oils. Medium-chain triglyceride (MCT) oil is a type of saturated fatty acid. MCT oil can provide many medical benefits and it aids in managing ketosis. MCT oil can be quickly converted into ketone bodies, making it an excellent and efficient source of energy.

What Not to Eat

If you are going to do a strict, clean, ketogenic diet regimen, all processed and refined foods should be eliminated from your diet. A general rule of thumb is if it comes in a ready-made, pre-packaged container then it should be avoided at all costs. If you did not make something from "scratch" then it is most likely something that you should avoid consuming. Now if you choose to allow yourself a "cheat meal" or "cheat day" then you may take in some processed carbohydrates on this day as will be discussed later.

Here is a list of some foods you should reduce or eliminate:

- boxed cereal
- cakes
- candy
- cookies

- conventional diary
- ice cream
- juices
- junk foods
- pasta

- pizza
- soft drinks
- store bought desserts
- table sugar
- white flour

Beverages

Diet soft drinks are perfectly acceptable and may be consumed as long as they are calorie-free.   So, what about that study that said diet drinks are bad and will cause you to gain more weight than drinking sugary soft drinks? Well, to set the record straight, the studies stating that diet drinks are bad are from epidemiological studies, which look to find a correlation between 2 things for future studies.   Basically, these studies have shown the correlation that unhealthy people drink diet soda.   From there, it was suggested that diet drinks are no better than regular soft drinks. Bit of a stretch isn't it? Better designed studies have not shown any correlation with diet drinks and health risks. In fact, diet drinks have not been shown to affect insulin levels or to inhibit fat loss. So, for now, if a diet drink is going to help you make it through the day, have at it. Just make sure that whatever you are drinking is calorie or at least sugar free.

Alcohol

If you are going to implement a ketogenic diet it is recommended that you do not consume any alcohol. Alcohol can work against a ketogenic diet by gradually slowing down the weight loss process. This occurs because alcohol is a toxin and is burned before anything else. Your body must process it and your weight loss efforts will stall when you do consume it. If you do choose to consume alcohol, it is very important that you look up information concerning the nutritional facts.

When it comes to beer, try choosing a lighter beer over the regular types of beer because they generally tend to have fewer calories and carbohydrates. Make no mistake, most forms of beers contain a high amount of carbohydrates so if possible, choose not to consume beer.

Wine is better to consume than beer, 5 fluid ounces of wine has approximately 4-5 grams of total net carbohydrates. Just because the net carbohydrates for wine is low does not mean that wine can be consumed daily. Wine should be consumed in moderation and only on occasion. Choose dry white wines and dry red wines as well as champagne that has no flavors or sweeteners added.

If you are going to choose alcohol, go with the hard liquors. These will most likely have zero grams of net carbohydrates when they contain no added flavors or sweeteners. Elect for whiskey, vodka, gin, rum, and tequila when determining what type of liquor to purchase.

Milk

Milk contains around 12 grams of carbohydrates in 8 fluid ounces. This is a high number of carbohydrates, especially for your low-carb days. If you are going to consume milk, use milk that is unpasteurized and contains the full amount of fat. It is, however, highly recommended that milk be avoided on a ketogenic diet. Whenever possible choose an alternative type of milk over the conventional type of milk.

Chapter 7: Additional Tips for Success

Tip #1: Drink a lot of water!!!

Water is already a key factor in everyday life but it becomes even more important when you start a ketogenic diet. For roughly the first two weeks after beginning a ketogenic diet, you will most likely experience some common side effects due to your body adapting to a ketogenic diet. Among these side effects are dehydration, constipation, and cramps. These generally can be relieved with an increased intake of water. Drinking more water will also increase your urine production which is important in getting rid of toxins from the body.

Most significantly, water contains absolutely no calories which is wonderful because you will be needing those calories elsewhere. Water also has the benefit of being a natural appetite suppressant. This will be most useful when you feel hungry in between meals. As a general rule of thumb when it comes to any diet; if you feel hungry in between meals, you should drink some water.

You can use fruits and vegetables to flavor water if needed to make the taste more palatable. A note to remember: if you want to use ingredients to flavor your water, be sure to include the carbohydrate counts of these ingredients in your daily total carbohydrate count.

Here is a list of common ingredients used to flavor water:

- cucumbers
- cherries
- ginger
- grapefruit

- kiwi
- lavender
- lemons
- limes
- mangoes
- mint
- oranges
- peaches
- pineapples
- raspberries
- rosemary
- strawber-ries
- watermel-on

It is important to note that you can drink any calorie free drink to meet your fluid requirements. Although it is important to drink more water, you may also drink coffee, diet drinks, tea, and sugar free sports drinks. As mentioned earlier, propel and powerade zero are crucial to replenishing electrolytes.

Tip #2: Keep a journal or diary

When first starting a ketogenic diet, you should use a diet journal or at least a program to keep track of your total daily requirements of calories, carbohydrates, protein, and fats. The easiest way to keep track of these numbers is for you to keep a log of them somewhere. This is especially important if you are using a keto diet for weight loss. At some point during your diet, you will hit a plateau and your weight loss will stall. This is normal and happens with any diet. If you have kept a good log, you will be able to adjust your diet by increasing or decreasing the amount of carbohydrates, protein, and fats you consume each day.

Keeping a journal or diary can also be useful when you start to incorporate new foods as well as eliminate foods. It can also double as a cheat sheet for your meal plans and recipes. It is highly recommended that you record everything when you start your diet. This will help you to look back and figure out what things were successful as well as those that did not work out quite as well for you. By keeping track of everything when you first start your diet, your journal will become an invaluable tool to assist you with your progression of ketogenic dieting.

Tip #3: Try to be as strict as possible

This is probably the hardest step of keto dieting because it takes the most dedication, discipline, and self-restraint. Eliminating carbohydrates is very hard, especially in the beginning.   However, as you get fat adapted and get through the first couple of weeks, you will find that you don't crave the sugary refined foods the way you used to. You'll feel so much better without these foods and when you eat them again, you'll feel sick afterwards. So, if you can make it the first few weeks, you will be successful.

In order to resist temptation and get through those first couple of hard weeks, it is important to be prepared. First off, get rid of the junk food in your cabinets and refrigerator and stock them with only foods appropriate for your ketogenic diet. It is hard not to eat that snack that you know is waiting for you in the cabinet. This is especially true on those days when you seem to be hungry despite eating all your planned-out meals. This is when only buying what you plan on eating becomes important.

It is crucial that you make a list of foods that you need for the week. It is recommended to try to do this on a weekly basis. If you do not need it, do not buy it. It is a simple concept but it can be difficult to follow.

Tips #4: Plan your meals for the week

This is ideally done before you buy your groceries so that you will know exactly what to buy. The first thing you need to do is figure out what your total carbohydrates, protein, and fat intake for the day should be. After you have each of those numbers for the day you can begin to formulate what you will prepare as your meals for the day. A meal plan for a low carbohydrate and high carbohydrate cheat day is shown as an example below.

Example meal:

Low-carbohydrate day:

- **Breakfast**: Eggs (made any way) with bacon and coffee with heavy cream
- **Morning snack**: .5 Avocado seasoned as desired
- **Lunch**: Quick tuna salad with mayo, tuna and seasonings wrapped in a large lettuce leaf. 1 cup chicken bone broth
- **Afternoon snack**: string cheese
- **Dinner**: Roasted chicken with cauliflower

High-carbohydrate cheat day:

- **Breakfast**: 1 cup oatmeal with walnuts, 0.50 cup blueberries, 1 cup almond milk
- **Morning snack**: banana and protein bar

- **Lunch**: 4 ounces tuna, 1 cup asparagus, orange
- **Afternoon snack**: apples with peanut butter, whey protein shake
- **Dinner**: 6 ounces of steak, 1 cup roasted bell peppers, 1 cup steamed cauliflower, 1 medium sweet potato

Tip #5: Use a variety of seasonings and spices

This is probably your best tool when it comes to preparing meals and changing the flavors of your foods. Depending on what you season some foods with, you can create completely new flavor profiles. This is especially helpful and significant when you are just starting out and creating new meal plans.

You should be mindful when choosing some seasonings and spices because they may contain sugars and carbohydrates. Be sure to check the nutritional facts and add the necessary amounts of carbohydrates to your overall total for the day.

Some of the more popular and common seasoning and spices that are used for ketogenic dieting include:

- basil
- black pepper
- cayenne pepper
- chili powder
- cilantro
- cinnamon
- cumin
- dill
- garlic
- ginger
- ginseng
- mustard seed
- oregano
- paprika
- parsley
- rosemary

- salt
- thyme
- turmeric

Tip #6: Sauces and condiments

When it comes to sauces and condiments it is best to create your own. However, there are options available if this is not possible or time consuming. Most mustards are ok to use as are a lot of hot sauces. Ketchup typically contains quite a bit of carbohydrate so if you can, stay away from it. If this is the only available sauce, try to choose a type of ketchup that has no added sugar and contains a small number of carbohydrates.

When it comes to salad dressings it is best to create your own. With a little bit of olive oil and balsamic vinaigrette, you can create a fast and easy salad dressing. Just remember that if you do purchase store-bought salad dressing, you should choose options that have full fat. These types of dressings should most likely be consumed on your high-carbohydrate cheat days so they do not end up working against you.

BBQ sauce should be completely avoided at all costs, they contain a large amount of sugar. Mayonnaise is an option as it is pure fat. When choosing a type of relish, go with the option that contains no added sugar and be wary of the carbohydrate content. Most sugar substitutes may be used, as well as sauces that are made with sugar substitutes. As with everything else, read the labels and check the carbohydrate contents of anything you decide to use.

Tip #7: The egg is your friend

The egg is arguably one of the most diverse types of food because it can be prepared in several ways and can be consumed at any time of the day. The egg is a natural and excellent source of protein and contains many nutrients.

Here is a list of potential benefits of the egg:

- inexpensive
- may promote weight loss
- essential for maintaining muscle mass and building lean muscle mass
- contains roughly 6 grams of protein, and 13 essential minerals and vitamins
- may aid in vision health, a healthy pregnancy, weight management, brain function, and muscle strength

- aids in reducing hunger

Here is a list of ways an egg can be prepared:

- baked eggs
- deviled eggs
- eggnog
- egg salad
- frittata
- hard boiled
- omelet
- over easy
- poached
- soft boiled
- scrambled
- sunny side up
- quiche

Tip #8: Use Alternative Flours

If you choose to use these products, it is recommended that you use them on your high-carbohydrate days because they typically have a higher number of carbohydrates. There are great alternatives for regular flour and can be used for recipes involving desserts and baking. This is great for those individuals who choose to implement "cheat meals" or "cheat days".

You can still consume some of your favorite type of desserts and baking goods, you just have to be more mindful of the ingredients that you use. Baking with these alternative flours does take some getting used to, as they will commonly call for various amounts of liquids compared to conventional flour.

Tip #9: Supplements

Depending on why you chose to incorporate ketogenic dieting, you may want to consider adding a few supplements to ensure you are covering your nutritional bases and to maximize your results. To get the greatest results, you should take a multivitamin, a greens supplement, and a fiber supplement.

The first supplement you should consider taking on this diet is a multivitamin and mineral supplement. A vitamin is an organic compound that is needed in trace amounts in the body to perform important regulatory functions. Vitamins play a role in digestion, energy transfer, growth, nervous system function, and much more. Minerals, like vitamins, are needed by the body and act as building blocks for body structures, cofactors in enzymatic reactions, enzymes, and as electrolytes (which are responsible for such things as muscle contraction, nerve impulses, and fluid balance). Vitamins and minerals must be obtained from the diet and a well-balanced diet can provide all of these required elements that you need. With this diet, we need to ensure we are still getting these essential vitamins so a multivitamin and mineral supplement is essential.

The second essential supplement that is recommended is a greens supplement. This supplement is a blend of veggies, fruits, algae, and grasses that have been compacted into a powdered form. This supplement will help provide the nutrition that is lacking from a diet low in fruits and vegetables. If you consistently consume 10 or more servings of fruits and vegetables daily, you'll likely not need a greens supplement. However, we know that may not be the case with this diet. Even with conventional dieting or diets, studies show that most people miss that mark. Supplementation with greens supplements can benefit energy, recovery, antioxidant status, and bone health. Consuming adequate fruits and veggies appear to reduce cardiovascular disease, high blood cholesterol, osteoporosis, type 2 diabetes, high blood pressure, obesity, stroke, asthma, and various cancers. So, add a greens supplement daily to the list so that you are not missing out on these benefits. These can be found at most supermarkets in a low-calorie powder form or capsule that has fiber and probiotics so pick one up.

If you aren't eating enough greens, then you should supplement with a fiber supplement. It is crucial to make sure that you are getting enough fiber to keep you regular and for good GI health. If you are eating plenty of green veggies, then you should be fine. However, if you are just supplementing a greens supplement and not eating much or any veggies, you should be taking a fiber supplement. Twenty-five grams of fiber a day is the absolute minimum you should be getting for optimal health. Therefore, it may be prudent to take a supplement in order to get at least this minimum amount. The best way to get additional fiber is by using a bulk powder like sugar-free Benefiber or Metamucil. Benefiber is often preferred as it is essentially tasteless and can mix in any liquid. This will add a few calories to your day but will not impact your diet since it's all coming from mostly undigested fibrous carbohydrates. Stay away from fiber gummies and tablets as these tend to have added sugars and are overall less in fiber.

Tip #10: Know Your Goal and Achieve It

Have measurable and specific goals to keep you on track. This is more important when using ketogenic diet for weight loss but it can help your dietary compliance no matter what your goals are.

First off, have a realistic main goal that you want to accomplish. This should have a set time frame that you want to accomplish it in and it should be something you can measure. For instance, if you want to get leaner and lose weight, you main goal may be to lose 20 pounds in 2 months. This is a specific goal and it's measurable. It's important that you pick a goal that is realistic as well.

Once you have a goal in mind, write it down and ensure that you are making weekly strides toward this goal. Personally, I write my main goal and weekly goals down on an index card and monitor my results every week to make sure I am following through on the game plan. If I wanted to lose 20 pounds in 2 months, I'd write on my index card that I will lose 20 pounds by such and such date exactly 2 months from the current day. Then I'd write my first weekly goal out. It would be I will lose 3 pounds by that upcoming Saturday. I'd write down my current weight and make sure I was losing weight appropriately through the week to ensure I met my weekly goal that Saturday. Once I measured my weight on Saturday, I would set a new goal for the following week based on my previous week's results. This would ensure that I was staying on track and doing everything I needed to do to reach my ultimate goal of dropping 20 pounds in a month.

You should think about why you want to a ketogenic diet before you choose to start one. Your decision as to why you want to accomplish your goal will be your motivation throughout the process. This motivation will be what gets you through the challenging times that you may experience while dieting. This is especially true for the first two weeks since this period is typically problematic for many individuals. Keep your eye on the prize and use your motivation to help you accomplish your goals.

Chapter 8: What is Intermittent Fasting?

So what is intermittent fasting and why should you be using it? Intermittent fasting has been around forever as people have been using it for thousands of years as a means of achieving a higher consciousness or communing with a higher power. More recently, however, it has been gaining popularity for its ability to allow people to get lean, build more muscle mass, and obtain health benefits that sound like science fiction.

The most basic form of intermittent fasting requires practitioners to skip breakfast before going on to eat regularly throughout the day. This unrestrictive diet plan is a terrific choice for those who find sticking to traditional diet plans practically impossible as it requires fewer changes to your diet overall while still producing noticeable results almost from the start. Many users find success via intermittent fasting in both the short and the long-term because it is relatively easy to stick with, once you get used to it, while still providing results comparable to more traditional diet plans.

The reason that intermittent fasting is so useful comes from the basic fact that the body behaves quite differently when it is in a fed state compared to when it is in a fasting state. A fed state is any period where the body is currently absorbing nutrients from foods it is actively digesting. This state begins roughly 5 minutes after you have finished a meal and generally lasts for about 5 hours depending on the type of foods you consumed. While your body is thus occupied, it is also creating insulin which signals your body to store the food it has taken in as body fat or glycogen. During this time, it is impossible to burn fat as your body is in storage mode.

Once digestion has finished, the body enters a buffer period that can last up to 12 hours depending on what was eaten last and personal digestive differences. It takes the body this long to process the insulin that was created after the last meal and get back to the level it started from. Only after these levels have once again normalized will your body be able to move back into a fasting state in which it can burn fat as effectively as possible.

The significant period of time required to reach this fasting state means that most people will never go without eating long enough to experience its benefits. Instead, if you want to reach this ideal fat-burning state you need to alter your standard eating habits and break free of the 3 square meals a day mentality.

Intermittent fasting benefits

First and foremost, allowing your body to spend time in a fasting state will lead to a natural improvement in both weight loss and muscle gain but those are only the most obvious of intermittent fasting's many benefits. You will also find that you have significantly more time throughout the day when you remove both preparing and eating a meal from your schedule. Along similar lines, you will also find that you have more money in your food budget as you won't need to worry about costly breakfast foods. While giving up breakfast might sound difficult at first, with a little practice you will be surprised how easily you get into the habit.

In addition to padding out the time you have in the day, along with your bank account, intermittent fasting is also known to allow those who practice it to live longer, healthier lives. Studies show that spending time in a fasting state causes your body to expend less energy on processing food, energy which is then spent on reinforcing core survival processes in much the way that it does if you are starving. While your body might react to them in the same way, starving and fasting affect the body in dramatically different ways, however, which means you end up with a net positive result.

Furthermore, when your cells don't have to spend all of their time processing energy they break down more slowly which means that by practicing intermittent fasting you are ensuring that each and every part of you lives longer than it otherwise would. This, in turn, leads to a wide variety of benefits including a greatly reduced risk of cardiovascular disease and stroke. Intermittent fasting has even been proven to lessen the overall effects of chemotherapy on cancer patients. You don't need to practice intermittent fasting for a prolonged period of time to see these benefits either, they will start to manifest themselves as soon as you cut down on the number of calories you are consuming by as little as 15 percent.

Further improvements include enhanced oxidative resistance, kidney function and glucose tolerance as well as a boost to the reproductive organs and a decrease in blood pressure all from simply reducing the amount of stress that is placed on your system from eating three large meals every day. Intermittent fasting is also known to decrease your overall level of stress while enhancing the effectiveness of your digestive tract and several other major organs. It has even been proven to increase the effectiveness of the mitochondria in your cells, allowing them to utilize existing energy as effectively as possible. In turn, this enhances the cells resistance to oxidation damage which leads to a decrease in the risk of cancer.

Many types of intermittent fasting are also known to be medically approved when it comes to decreasing the risk of developing type 2 diabetes in those who are already suffering from the effects of pre-diabetes. It has been shown to reduce glucose levels back to an acceptable range in as little as 1 year.

Fasting is also known to induce beneficial hormonal changes, in addition to reducing insulin production it is also known to increase the production of adrenalin, nor-adrenalin, and human growth hormone (HGH). These hormones are released in times of stress such as fasting, exercise, or a fight/flight situation. The release of adrenalin and noradrenalin cause an increase in alertness and the breakdown of fat in the body to provide energy to go out and deal with the stressful situation, be it to fight for survival or hunt for food. The stimulatory effects of adrenalin and noradrenalin allow many people to benefit from an increase in concentration and alertness during their fast. The increase in HGH is another huge benefit with intermittent fasting. You don't have to do like Sylvester Stallone and inject HGH to benefit, all you have to do is fast. As HGH is suppressed when the body is in a fed state, it stands to reason that production spikes during fasting. In fact, a 24 hour fast will typically result in a 2.5 increase in HGH response in the body.

This increase in HGH provides people with numerous benefits. Most notably, an increase in HGH will result in more fat burning and the prevention of muscle loss during the fast. HGH does this by increasing the amount of fat being burned by the body as fuel and reducing the body's need for glucose. By decreasing the body's need for glucose, it prevents muscle from being broken down to provide this glucose. It's important to realize that in order to get this crucial HGH release and burn fat while preserving muscle mass, you must be fasting and that's a huge benefit to intermittent fasting over traditional dieting.

While these real, measurable health benefits are plenty reasons to give intermittent fasting a try, what many practitioners ultimately find most enjoyable about the process is that it offers up additional mental clarity as well. Additionally, it is so easy to practice that virtually anyone can adjust to the process with very little effort. So much so that studies have found that even those who were extremely overweight and had already had difficulty sticking to any type of diet were routinely able to stick with it for 3 months or more, much longer than they had been able to with many more restrictive diets. Even better, while they were on an intermittent fasting-based diet they saw just as much weight loss as those who stuck to much more complicated diet plans. Finally, after 12 months of intermittent fasting they had managed to lose more weight overall than any of the other dieters in the study.

My favorite benefit of intermittent fasting is its ability to increase satiety and curb hunger. This may sound paradoxical since it's logical that going without food will just increase your hunger. However, by going without food, your body starts to produce appetite suppressing catecholamines. You'll find that if you stay busy and ignore your initial hunger pangs, you will be less hungry throughout the day. When you do finally eat, you be able to eat a larger meal than you would had you been eating throughout the day and still maintain the same calorie allotment. This is a plus for me as I'm a big eater. I would rather eat two 1000 calorie meals than four 500 calorie meals. These larger meals are more satiating and can definitely help with hunger when you are in a calorie deficit.

Basics of fasting

While intermittent fasting isn't that complicated, there are a handful of rules that you are going to want to keep in mind in order to get the most out of the process. It is important to stick with them rigorously in order to see real results in a reasonable period of time.

Burn more calories than you take in: While burning more calories than you consume is a core tenant of many diets, it is crucial when it comes to intermittent fasting as it can be very easy to overeat once you have broken your fast, unintentionally negating all of your hard work. Don't use your fast as a reason to reward yourself with an extra large meal or eat more than you would usually. By the time you end you fast, you should have burned up quite a bit of fat but this can be put right back on just as easily if you eat more calories than you expended throughout the day. The best policy is to eat a regular sized meal or a meal that fits within your daily caloric allotment for fat loss if that is your goal. Remember that there are 3,500 calories in a pound which means that every week you are going to need to create this much of a deficit if you hope to lose at least one pound a week.

Control yourself: In order to fast effectively, you need to have the self-control to ensure that you can go without eating for at least 12 hours at a time, on a regular basis. Any calories consumed during this time will reset the insulin regulation cycle and force your body out of its maximum fat-burning state. Ideally you will want to consume a calorie deficit of 500 calories per day if you hope to see at least one pound of weight lost per week.

Keep it up: When it comes to making a habit out of intermittent fasting, it is crucial that you stick with it long enough for your body to get used to the process. At first, you may feel like you're starving out. You're going to think about food and about how hard it is to fast. However, anytime a craving or thought about food comes to mind, just push it out and focus on something else. You'll find that this feeling of starvation quickly dissipates and your hunger will go away. In fact, you'll find that you have more energy and more productive days while fasting.

Chapter 9: Types of Fasting

4:3 and 5:2 Method

With this intermittent fasting plan, you eat a regular healthy diet for either 4 or 5 days and then for the remaining days you only eat somewhere between 500 and 600 calories. The baseline average caloric intact is 2,500 calories for men and 2,000 calories for women. Some famous names that swear by this diet are former UK Prime Minister Davide Cameron and actress Jennifer Aniston. The point with both plans is to not feel deprived on the days that you are free to eat normally, just be sure to do so in moderation and don't allow yourself to over-indulge.

Health benefits from this type of inter-mittent fasting plan include increased insulin resistance among those with dia-betes, reduction in heart arrhythmias, relief from hot flashes caused by menopause and relief from asthma and seasonal allergies. Additionally, a 12-week study of those using the 4:3 method revealed that the average practi-tioner saw a reduction in fat mass by 7.7 pounds with no negative impact to mus-cle mass and an overall body weight re-duction of 11 pounds. They also saw a reduction in negative cholesterol along with lower levels of blood pressure and a 20 percent reduction in triglycerides.

Furthermore, they saw their leptin levels decrease 40 percent (which means they were less hungry overall). Finally, they experienced a significant reduction in levels of CRP which is used as a marker for general levels of inflammation in the body.

4:3 Differences

The 4:3 plan is more restrictive than the 5:2 plan simply because you get to eat less overall throughout the week. This means you are going to want to more closely limit the amount of refined, sugary or processed foods that you consume on the days you eat full meals simply because your body will then crave additional fatty acids on the days you are fasting which will make the experience more difficult.

It is important not to overindulge on the days that you are eating freely as it can be easy to go over your calorie limit and defeat the purpose of the entire exercise. With time, you can train your body to expect a well-structured diet and you won't feel as hungry during the fast days. The 4:3 plan also recommends that you skip breakfast and measure your weight daily. For those whose weight tends to fluctuate more than average this is not recommended, however, as it can be disheartening.

Tips for success

The following are ways to manage this type of intermittent fasting, but be aware that your fasting days should include as few carbohydrates as possible for the best effect.

Experiment with meal time: During the days you are fasting you may find it easier to subsist on 500 or 600 calories if you mix up the time at which you eat. Most people are less hungry in the morning so it might help to push back the time you eat some of your calories until later in the day. Likewise, instead of eating 3 meals where you only consume 200 calories at a time, you may find it helpful to simply eat two 300 calorie meals instead. Eating a late brunch at 11 am and then consuming the rest of your calories around 7 or 8 pm has proven to be more effective for many people.

Minimize calories but maximize flavor: Soups are a great way to extend your caloric intake out as much as possible. Research into this type of fasting has shown that a vegetable soup can keep those fasting feeling fuller for an extra 2 hours compared to those who consume the same caloric amount of vegetables alone. When you make your soups, don't skimp on the seasonings as well, as long as they don't include many carbs. Vinegar and lemon juice on salads is a fine choice, as are chili flakes or curry pastes in soups, stews and with baked beans. A good meal composition for these days is two meals composed primarily of vegetables with a small serving of protein such as tofu, lean meat, eggs or fish.

Strive for fresh ingredients: Seasonal products will ensure that you keep a good amount of variety in your diet. They will also help your wallet as they are going to be cheaper than other options while also being healthier as well.

During the winter months, good choices are parsnip and butternut squash, try them in a soup or roasted with a low-fat feta cheese. If you are feeling up to a taste challenge, you can try some peppers (red or green) that have been cut in half and stuffed with tuna cream cheese or eggs and then grilled.

Additional fasting day foods that you will learn to love include natural yogurt and berries, boiled and baked eggs, cauliflower, tomato and miso soup and grilled fish or other lean meats. When it comes to beverages you are going to want to stick with water (sparkling or still) and plenty of black coffee or tea. Black coffee is the best choice because the caffeine will naturally serve as an appetite suppressant. It is also a diuretic so it will help you lose weight more reliably as well. If you lead a busy lifestyle, you can cheat once in a while with a prepackaged meal that is low in calories but this shouldn't become a regular part of your diet.

Sample meal plan

Breakfast: Skip it. If you enjoy a morning meal then you will need to eliminate the snack during the day. You may also skip lunch instead.

Lunch: Lentil, leek or chicken soup with a small snack such as a tangerine.

Dinner: A small portion of fish or fillet of grilled chicken with a side salad with lemon juice and seasonings as dressing.

Snack: Carrot sticks to fill out the remainder of your calories.

Chapter 10: Eat-Stop-Eat Method

With this type of intermittent fasting method, you eat normally 5 days a week and then fast for either 20 or 24 hours the other 2 days. For example, you would eat dinner on Tuesday, fast until dinner time Wednesday, and then resume regular eating on Thursday. You will want to schedule your fasting days at least 2 days apart from one another to give your body time to recover from the strain of not eating for 24 hours.

On the days that you are fasting, you will want to limit yourself to water, diet soda, tea and coffee. You'll end your fast with a regular sized meal. Make sure when you do, that you do not binge on food. Eat a regular sized meal or slightly more than a normal sized meal but ensure you do not allow yourself to use fasting as an excuse for gluttony. If you over consume you daily allotment of calories after your fast, you will undo a lot of your progress. On the days you are eating regularly you are going to want to feel free to eat what you will, within reason.

Some people will not be able to adapt to such a strict type of fasting, you will know that it is not for you if you continue being irritable during fast days after a month or so and if you continue to experience periods of dizziness or headaches. With that being said, the benefits to this intermittent fasting method are undeniable and it offers the freedom to alter when you are fasting based on need.

Whatever you do, however, it is important to never fast for 2 consecutive days and never fast for more than 2 days in a single week.

Watch your fluid intake: As this method of intermittent fasting is extremely strict, it is very important that you remain hydrated while you are fasting. This is crucial not only because it will help you to deal with the lack of food, but also because fasting in this fashion is sure to dehydrate you more than normal. An optimal way of checking your hydration status is by monitoring the color of your urine output. If you are sufficiently hydrated, your urine should be lightly straw colored to clear in appearance. If you urine is dark, you should be drinking more fluids.

Additional tips: When utilizing this method of intermittent fasting it is crucial that you maintain your self-control when you have finished fasting and don't let yourself fall into the habit of fasting and then bingeing. This will cause havoc within your system and lead to poorer results overall. This means that this type of intermittent fasting is only for those who have stalwart self-control.

On the days that you are not fasting you may want to practice resistance-style weight training to boost effectiveness. Likewise, on the days that you are fasting, you can do yoga or cardio. A session of cardio will suppress your appetite and make it easier to continue the fast. Hit a cardio session on a treadmill, elliptical, or other means when you are feeling hungry or thinking of food and you'll stop hunger in its tracks. As well, you'll maximize your growth hormone release and burn more fat before you end your fast.

While practicing this type of fasting it is common to initially feel angry, fatigued, anxious and also experience periods of light-headedness or frequent headaches. These should fade in time, however, and if they don't you should discontinue this type of intermittent fasting and consult a physician.

Chapter 11: 16:8 Method

Also known as the Leangains protocol, this type of intermittent fasting requires that men fast for 16 hours per day and women fast for at least 14 hours per day while eating a reasonable amount for the remaining 8 or 10 hours. Actor Hugh Jackman is a big proponent of this type of intermittent fasting.

The Leangains method of intermittent fasting has been proven to lead to the most noticeable weight loss in the shortest period of time and proponents tout the fact that you are likely going to be sleeping for at least half of the period during which you will be fasting which makes the overall process much more manageable. During the time when you are not fasting each day, you can break your total calorie count up any way you like as long as you are still cutting out approximately 500 calories from your daily dietary needs and eating in a relatively health-conscious fashion. While you are in the fasting period of the day, you will need to restrict yourself to water, tea, black coffee and 0 calorie sodas.

For the best results for those who are either already overweight or have a mainly sedimentary lifestyle, cutting out most, if not all, starchy carbs from your diet is also recommended. It may be difficult at first to cram all of your caloric requirements into this time period, but it will get easier with time. Most practitioners of this type of intermittent fasting either split their calories between 2 extra-filling meals or between 3 regular-sized meals and you should try both to see which works best for you. Whatever you decide on, it is important to keep in mind that consistency is very important to your long-term success.

A study done by the Obesity Society found that the most effective fasting period is between 10 pm and 2 pm, for men, and 12 am and 2 pm for women. Having your first meal at 2 pm has been shown to reduce feelings of hunger for the rest of the day while also maximizing fat burned throughout the entire day as well.

Of all the types of intermittent fasting, the 16:8 model is the one that can be most easily adapted to fit any schedule. What's more, 2 large meals in either 8 or

10 hours is enough to keep most people going strong for about 12 hours which means you will really only need to allow your body to adjust to 4 hours without the fuel it is craving. A common pattern for many practitioners is to eat a large and filling dinner at around 7 pm and then fast until lunch the next day. This will allow you to eat at a normal time and fit intermittent fasting into an average office job schedule. Nevertheless, you are really free to break your fast as early in the day as you like as long as you stop eating early enough in the day to repeat the cycle successfully.

If you find that you are having a difficult time getting started with, and sticking to, this plan then it may be because you are striving to force an ineffective eating schedule onto yourself. It is important to

consider the timeframe that will make it
as easy to go without eating for a prolonged period of time as possible as opposed to one that you have to struggle
with for the full 16 hours. Once you do
find a timeframe that works for you, it is
important to lock it in as much as possible as this will help your body adjust and
allow you to see the greatest amount of
success possible.

If you end up finding yourself really
struggling with the final few hours of the
fast then you are likely not consuming
enough protein during the times when
you are eating. During this span, you are
going to want to focus on consuming at
least 55 grams of protein for women and
60 grams for men. This is important not
only to keep you feeling sated through-

out your fast but also when it comes to building strong muscles.

This type of intermittent fasting is also great for those who enjoy exercising regularly as you are still consuming food regularly enough to not have to alter your exercise regimen a noticeable amount. If this is the case for you, it is important to always break your fast with lots of protein along with nuts, dark green leafy vegetables and seeds. When consumed in tandem they are sure to provide you with the energy you need to make it through the day. Keeping your energy levels at an appropriate level can be tricky but it is definitely something you are going to need to focus on in order to ensure that your body doesn't falter under the additional strain.

It is recommended that you break your fast with a medium-sized meal before exercising in a four-hour window and then eating another larger meal after you have finished exercising. During this secondary meal, you are going to want to be sure to eat plenty of complex carbohydrates that ensure you have enough fuel to keep yourself going for a full 14 to 16 hours. Only by making a concentrated effort to fuel up properly will you be able to stick to this schedule effectively in the long run.

If you plan on exercising some days and not on others then you will need to take this disparity into account as well and vary the number of calories and carbs you are consuming accordingly to ensure that you aren't accidentally overeating. On the days you don't plan on exercising you are going to want to maintain your daily weight loss by consuming about 60 percent of your daily caloric total during your first meal and then split the remaining calories between either one or two additional meals.

Chapter 12: Warrior Method

If you are looking for an intermittent fasting variant that is between the 16:8 method and the eat, stop, eat method then the warrior method has you covered. For this type of intermittent fasting, you spend 20 hours of the day fasting and then consume your daily caloric requirements in the remaining 4 hours. The first meal you consume should include about 65 percent of your daily caloric intake and the second should take up the remaining 35 percent.

The basis for this type of intermittent fasting comes from the idea that ancient humans hunted at night which meant they spent a majority of their time in a fasting state. This fact leads proponents of the warrior method to posit that the human body is more poised to absorb nutrients properly by simply eating in a condensed window at the end of the day. The idea here is that by eating during this window you will end up feeling fuller while still consuming a smaller number of calories overall.

While this might sound like a bit of a stretch, the science behind it is surprisingly sound. You see, every night when the sun goes down, this transition causes the human body's fight or flight response to activate because the lack of readily available light means it is more difficult to identify threats. This change is felt throughout the body and one of the side effects is that you will naturally burn more fat from the foods you eat during this time.

For those who feel as though they won't be able to go 20 hours between meals, the warrior diet actually allows for 1 serving of dark, leafy green vegetables as well as 30 grams of protein. The best way to take advantage of this fact is to consume the vegetables prior to exercising and the protein afterwards to give you extra energy and help you build muscles, respectively. When you do finally break your fast, it is important that you do so with a meal that contains lots of healthy vegetables as well as an equal mix of healthy fats, complex carbohydrates and lean protein.

However, it is important that you consume them in the proper order for the greatest benefits. First you will want to eat your vegetables, followed by your protein, followed by your healthy fats and then finish the meal with your complex carbohydrates. This will allow your body to process everything as efficiently as possible and also give you the fuel you need to make it 20 hours between meals. This combination will also allow your body to repair itself more easily, which is important if you plan to exercise regularly while practicing this form of intermittent fasting.

If you aren't in a position to exercise in the middle of the day for your snack, you are going to want to exercise in between your 2 meals for the best results. You are going to want to eat your first meal, wait an hour, exercise and then consume your second meal. While you will need to work on your timing to get everything done in just 4 hours, it will get easier with practice.

While it might seem extreme at first, the warrior method is actually one of the most popular ways of intermittent fasting due to its level of flexibility and for the fact that it allows for a snack. This relative freedom also makes it a great type of intermittent fasting to start with for novices while still being effective enough that experts may want to give it a try and will be able to do so fairly easily. Those who find it the most difficult are going to be folks who have very busy schedules that would prevent them from getting everything done in the short period of time that is required.

Prior to starting, it is important to keep in mind the way in which it can possibly affect your social life, which will be a turnoff for some people. Others may just not like having to eat their foods in a specific order which is crucial if you want to experience the full effects of the warrior diet method.

Chapter 13: Alternative Types of Intermittent Fasting

Forever fat loss

The forever fat loss type of intermittent fasting combines aspects of several different intermittent fasting methods to form something rather unique. What's more, you even get a cheat day from a more traditional diet each and every week. To balance out this cheat day, however, immediately following it you are not allowed to consume anything save water, diet soda, black coffee, tea and 0 calorie gum for 36 hours. You are also allowed to eat a single serving of dark, leafy green vegetables after 18 hours. The remaining days of the week are then split between the 16:8 method and the warrior method.

Fasting for 36 hours straight is automatically going to make this type of intermittent fasting off limits for some people as going without food for that long will really test the willpower of most people. Furthermore, the variety of the days means that you are going to need to have a semi-flexible schedule to account for the various differences. Additionally, you are going to need to limit your physical exercise to a minimum on your long fast day in order to get through it successfully.

When you make it to the end of your long fast, you are going to want to start with just a small meal to ensure you aren't overeating and also to get your digestive processes moving naturally after the absence of food. If you find that you have a difficulty controlling yourself during the fast, or that you feel the need to eat a large meal when you break your fast as opposed to a small one then this is likely not the most efficient form of fasting for you. You goal when fasting, regardless of the type of intermittent fasting that you chose, is to find a healthy and long-term dietary plan which means that if any part of the process causes you to act in an unhealthy fashion then you need to check yourself or focus on a different intermittent fasting method instead.

If you have the self-control and time to follow through, however, the results from the forever fat loss method are known to be the most significant of all the various types of intermittent fasting that are appropriate to undertake on a full-time basis. If you plan on following through with this type of intermittent fasting, then it is especially important to take extra care and ensure that your overall caloric intake and nutritional standards stay where they need to be through the standard warrior, 16:8 fasts, and the long fast. With so many different requirements between the various plans, it is very important that you make a calendar and stick with it to avoid losing a week's worth of progress simply because you got your plans mixed up for a few days. More importantly, it will help to ensure you stay within nutritional guidelines and don't cause yourself more harm than good in the process.

Alternate fasting

If you don't think you can go a full 12 hours without eating without worrying that you are going to pass out from hunger, then you may have more luck with the alternative fasting method. With this method, you simply eat normally 50 percent of the time and on the alternating days you cut your total caloric intake back to just 20 percent of your daily total. As such, you will still be able to generate the 3,500-calorie deficit required for one pound of weight loss without having to fast in a more tradi-tional sense.

The biggest downside to this type of in-termittent fasting is that you don't get the benefits of entering a true fasted state. However, limiting your calories is still going to help you moderate your weight more easily while also helping you get in the habit of restricting your diet. This will put you in a spot where you can more easily control your eating habits with a more traditional form of fasting in the future. If you are unsure of just how many calories you are consuming in a given day, it is important to always err on the side of consuming less than consuming more as hitting this 20 percent is key to seeing weight loss results. With that being said, it is important to hone in on just how many calories you need as perpetually consuming too few calories can lead to malnutrition which can, in turn, lead to long lasting bodily damage.

On your low-calorie days, you are going to want to make those calories stretch as far as possible, one common way of doing so is to find a protein powder that you like and use protein shakes to help you feel full without consuming all of your calories in one fell swoop. This is only a good way to get started, however, as natural, whole foods are always going to provide better results overall than artificial products.

A large number of people find this a very easy way to practice a variation of intermittent fasting in the long-term. So much so that it has nearly twice as many long-term adherents than any other type of intermittent fasting. What's more, you will likely see as much as 3 pounds of weight loss per week as your body transitions to this new way of eating.

Irregular fasting

If what you have read so far has you interested in intermittent fasting but you don't think you are ready to commit to anything long term then you may want to start out by simply fasting now and then for 12 hours or more at a given stretch, just to see how your body responds to the process. While this won't provide you with the weight loss or additional health benefits of committing to it on a regular basis, it will still give you a reasonable idea of what to expect from the process and if your body can handle the stress involved.

The key to success with irregular intermittent fasting is to not think of it as an either-or proposition. Every time you go at least 12 hours without eating you win and the more frequently you do so, the healthier you will be overall. Furthermore, if you practice this type of intermittent fasting for a long enough period of time then it is increasingly likely that you will develop the mental and physical discipline to move on to one of the more committed types of fasting as well. It doesn't matter how long it takes or if you start and stop repeatedly before making the switch, the only thing you have to lose from the process is unwanted weight.

Chapter 14: Incorporating IF with Ketogenic diet

Now that we have talked about different fasting strategies, we need to talk about how to incorporate these strategies along with ketogenic dieting in order to optimize our results.

First off, any of the intermittent fasting techniques described above can be utilized along with a keto diet to speed your results, get into ketosis faster, and attain better overall health. To incorporate intermittent fasting in a keto diet, simply ensure that you are hitting your macronutrient ratios and daily calorie allotment in your defined eating window, whatever that may be. It's really that simple. You'll attain all the physiological benefits from fasting and reach ketosis so much faster if you are not already in this metabolic state. If you are, then you'll be burning through fat faster than you ever thought possible and faster than possible with either dieting strategy alone. Although you can utilize the other methods of intermittent fasting, I find it prudent and easier to utilize the eat-stop-eat method and 16-8 methods of fasting. In the following sections, I will describe ways to utilize these methods and the ways I personally use them to get the best possible results.

Supercharged results with EAT-STOP-EAT

Utilizing the EAT-STOP-EAT method can supercharge your way to weight loss and get you back in to ketosis in record time. There are 2 great times to utilize this method; to jump start your keto-genic diet or to cut additional calories for the the week. I'll discuss when to use the two options in further detail in the following paragraphs.

The first method should be the primary usage for the EAT-STOP-EAT method. This method will entail not eating for 24 hours in order to get into ketosis faster. By not eating for 24 hours, you'll burn through any available glycogen faster and hit ketosis faster and maximize fat burning. This is a great way to jump start your ketogenic diet on the first day of your diet.

Another great way to use this method is with your cheat day planning. By utiliz-ing this method, you can also plan efficient cheat days. The problem with cheat days is that it's so easy to over-eat and completely erase all of your hard earned progress that you had worked so hard for the week before. This method of intermittent fasting can allow you to have your cake and eat it too. There's a couple of ways to incorporate this method to help you master your cheat day.

First off, you can use this intermittent fasting strategy by minimizing your possibility of cheat day damage. What do I mean by that? Well, if you are like me and are a voracious eater, you can completely undo a week's dieting progress by eating until you are sick on a planned cheat day. I've learned the hard way that a cheat day shouldn't be a planned day of seeing how much crap I can stuff down my throat. I've had cheat days where I would see if I could eat every single one of my favorite foods or snacks throughout the day and I'd usually succeed. However, I would be sick as hell that night and sorry for it the next day when I hopped on the scales or didn't make any progress the following week.

Here's how to minimize cheat day gluttony and still get great results. First off, plan a 24 hour day fast the day of your cheat day. Your last meal should be the only meal you eat on this day. Plan for your cheat day to be the end of the fast. Now, you can eat quite a bit and enjoy the foods that you had planned without overdoing it. Eat until you are satisfied and then stop. Don't gorge yourself. However, the great thing about this method is that even if you do gorge yourself, the one meal limitation will likely prevent you from overdoing it too badly. After your meal, you should be satisfied and done for the day. You should resume your diet the next day. If you want to get back into ketosis even faster, follow up your cheat meal with the next method.

The other method is to follow up your cheat day with a 24 hour fast the next day. This will enable you to burn up the glycogen you stored and get back into ketosis faster. You'll find that you will feel great fasting for 24 hours the day after a cheat meal or diet break. You'll have energy to burn and you'll be psychologically ready to get back after it. I find that I'm never hungry on these days and when I hit the gym, which I recommend doing right before ending the fast, I am stronger and more energetic.

This method can also be used when you hit a weight loss plateau. Sometimes, when dieting, you will need to reduce your calories further in order to continue making progress. This occurs for many different reasons. It generally happens as you lose weight and your daily maintenance level of calories decreases. This happens because a lighter body requires less energy to move itself and because your body become more efficient processing calories. So, you can take an additional 24 hour fast throughout the week to cut more calories and increase your weekly calorie deficit. This will get the scale moving again for you.

16-8 for Daily Excellence

The 16-8 method of intermittent fasting can be used daily and I personally use it daily. This method is great to allow you to benefit from daily fasting. I would recommend using this method daily if it fits your lifestyle. By incorporating this method daily, you will be able to increase your daily growth hormone release, build more muscle, burn more fat, and eat more satisfying meals.

This is how I use this method. By eating only twice a day after fasting for 16 hours, I can eat 2 large meals even during a calorie deficit. This works well for me as I am a big eater. By allowing myself 2 larger meals instead of smaller meals throughout the day, I am able to prevent hunger from getting the best of me and sabotaging my results. I will eat once at 2 PM and again at 9 PM after working out. This allow me to not feel hungry and to go to bed satisfied even during a calorie deficit.

Additional Tips

While each type of intermittent fasting is beneficial in its own way, they can also each be very complicated and difficult to stick with in both the long and the short term if you don't tackle them with the right mindset. The suggestions found in the following pages can make the process much easier, however, so it is recommended that you give them a try before throwing in the towel and going back to your old eating habits.

Stay true to yourself: While intermittent fasting can certainly provide you with a variety of healthy lifestyle changes, it doesn't mean it is going to be the right choice for everyone. While you should be able to make it through a number of fasts without slipping, once you have done so you are going to want to consider how difficult that period of time was for you. You will also need to consider what your natural habits are like when it comes to eating and what your overall relationship with food is like in general. It is important to keep in mind that intermittent fasting is not so much a diet as it is a lifestyle which means you should focus on long term success and not think about it as a short-term solution like you would most diets.

This long-term commitment is why you are going to want to seriously ask yourself if you are going to be able commit to fasting regularly in the long term, if not with the first type of intermittent fasting that you try then possibly the second or the third. Intermittent fasting should fit your lifestyle and make it easier for you to diet and incorporate your ketogenic diet.

Be aware of what your body is trying to tell you: While adjusting to intermittent fasting will almost always come with some side effects, it is important to remember that these are supposed to fade in time which means you are going to want to remain in touch with your body to ensure you don't end up hurting yourself in the process. If you find yourself experiencing longer or more severe symptoms it is important to stop immediately instead of powering through. Maintaining your overall health is key when it comes to maximizing the results from intermittent fasting and you can't do that if your body is reacting negatively to the process. Listen to the things your body is telling you and never try to push yourself past your limits. If you do, you could find yourself passing out from hunger, or worse.

Don't let yourself make excuses: While it is important to not get started on a new intermittent fasting plan when your schedule is extremely busy or you have extra stress or anxiety on your plate, it is also important to not keep putting it off every time something new comes up. Life is always going to be busy, that is why one of the benefits of intermittent fasting is having more time each fasting day. At some point, the reasons you have for putting it off are simply going to be excuses to avoid getting started. Be frank with yourself and understand that there is always going to be something standing in your way from making positive life changes. You simply need to power through it if you ever hope to see real success.

At some point, all you can do is say enough is enough and get down to business. After all, the only person that can really motivate you to stick with a healthy intermittent fasting diet plan in the long term is you. This is why it is so important to not let yourself down. If you truly commit to find personal success when it comes to your weight loss goals then there should be nothing that can stop you. It really is as simple as that.

Set the right goals: Once you do start your preferred intermittent fasting plan, you are going to want to take into account that a 3,500-calorie deficit is going to lead to the loss of one pound of fat, but that this equation doesn't take muscle growth into the equation at all. This means that if you are exercising regularly then you may end up losing less weight per week, but still end up looking and feeling better regardless. If you find yourself feeling discouraged based on the results from the scale, it is important to consider how long it took you to reach your current weight and fitness level and then give yourself a comparable period of time to get back to where you need to be. Getting to your current point didn't happen overnight and there is no reason to expect changing things up drastically will lead to overnight results either.

Start off the right way: If you have never gone without a meal for 12 hours in your life, then you are likely going to find the best results by starting with an intermittent fasting plan that limits when you eat to 12 hours a day and work your way up from there. It is important to take things slow and steady and to not push yourself too far too fast as you will likely experience side effects by doing so. Jumping right into a more serious type of intermittent fasting can lead to failure which can make it difficult to really give the process the fair shot it deserves.

If even 12 hours seems like a stretch, there is no reason you can't start with a more manageable timeframe and then work up from there. When you start intermittent fasting, you are not being judged based on how other people have found success. It is more about finding success for yourself and sticking to it in the long run, than meeting any specific goal, especially right out of the gate. Whatever you decide, it is important to try and stick with it as diligently as possible. Anything is an improvement over no weight loss plan at all.

Eat healthy: If, after giving yourself enough time to properly transition to an intermittent fasting diet, you still feel as though you are hungrier than it seems like you should be, you may want to consider the types of foods you are consuming and not just how many calories you are taking in each day. If you are eating a large amount of processed foods, then you are likely not actually getting the level of nutrition that your body needs in a day, especially when you take intermittent fasting into account. This means your body is burning through its available fuel faster than it should be. To counteract this development, simply add more healthy fats and lean protein to your diet. This should keep you feeling fuller for longer periods of time and make intermittent fasting much more manageable.

Consider the source of your hunger: While it may seem pretty straight forward, hunger is actually a common reaction to several different types of stimuli that may not actually have anything to do with your stomach and how empty it is. As such, assessing where your feelings of hunger are coming from can be a great way to address them without breaking your fast. Being dehydrated often results in feelings of hunger, as does nervousness, anxiety and sadness in some people. Once you have locked onto the reason for the hunger, you will likely find that it is much easier to deal with overall.

Don't settle for the first plan you try: The shear variety of different intermittent fasting plans available means that, even if you find the first plan you try easy to stick with, there might be a better one out there for you. Not trying multiple plans before you commit can cause you to lose out on something that is even better. After all, if there really isn't anything better out there for you then you can always come back around to your first choice and pick up where you left off. If you don't try them all, you'll never know. Of course, if you don't think you can last the full length of time then there is no point in pushing yourself past your tolerance level. Be aware of your limitations and choose accordingly.

Drink more water: While many people will naturally see this tip and assume that it means it is important to stay hydrated. In reality, it is a command to drink at least a gallon of water each and every day. This will not only help you to feel more sated while fasting, it will also ensure that your body continues to process toxins out of your system during the transitional phase when you are getting used to intermittent fasting. During this time, your body will effectively detoxify itself and rid itself of toxins as it adjusts to going without a full stomach all the time.

Additionally, this is good advice in general because a full 40 percent of all adults in the US are currently suffering from a mild state of dehydration without even knowing about it. This is especially perilous during a fasting state as your body doesn't have the tools to fight off the negative effects of this state as easily as it otherwise would. Remember, if you are feeling thirsty then it is already too late.

Keep busy: It doesn't matter if you are just getting started with intermittent fasting or if you have been doing it for months, keeping busy is a great way to keep your mind, and your body occupied when hunger sets in so that you can more easily ignore it and complete your fast successfully. Sitting around and thinking about the food that you will be eating when you break your fast is only going to make the time pass more slowly and leave you feeling hungrier as well.

Furthermore, you are going to want to make an effort to schedule all of your strenuous or difficult tasks either during the periods of time when you are free to eat, early on in a fast when you are still feeling somewhat full, or right at the end of your fast so that you can transition directly from the task to a nice, rewarding meal. Starting off a fast with unwanted tasks might not be entirely pleasant, but holding off on those tasks for an extended period of time is only going to make them more difficult to complete in the long run when you are having to dedicated more of your physical and mental energy to ignoring your hunger.

Schedule your time wisely: As long as you make it a point to schedule other activities around your fasting periods you will likely find that the fast doesn't interfere with your life at all once you get used to it. This means you will also want to consider periods where you may need to move the end of your fast up by as much as 2 hours. As long as you don't make a point of constantly shifting your fasting schedule you should find that this in no way negatively affects your overall results.

It is important to keep in mind that intermittent fasting is an extremely modular dietary plan which means you shouldn't feel trapped in your habit just because someone wants to make dinner plans at 8 pm and you don't normally break your fast until 9 pm. This is the case, of course, as long as you have the willpower to not let a small shift in your timeframe act as an excuse to let loose all self-control and either binge or give up on intermittent fasting entirely. As long as you can control yourself, a little variance now and then never hurt anybody.

Amino Acids: Branch chain amino acids (BCAA) are an important supplement to consider if you are planning on fasting for 24 hours or longer. They are useful in helping your body build muscle tissue while fasting while also promoting additional weight loss. It is important to procure some either online or from most health food stores prior to undertaking any fast of this length.

Chapter 15: Working Out with Keto and Fasting

How you workout during a ketogenic diet and how you structure your fasting intervals will all come down to your goals. It should be no question that you should be working out or exercising for optimal health. Why shouldn't you be? If you are interested in ketogenic dieting and fasting for health reasons, then you should also be utilizing exercise for its benefits as well. The fact that you can use intermittent fasting, ketosis, and exercise all together to augment weight loss should be logical but it is true that you can also use all of these to gain muscle mass as well. This section will give you strategies that you can use to optimize your fitness goals, no matter what they may be.

Weight Loss

So, it's pretty much intuitive that you can combine exercise with ketosis and intermittent fasting for weight loss. But, how should you combine this to maximize your results and ensure you are not damaging your health or hurting your progress? Can working out fasted hurt you? Will you burn up muscle mass if you do so?

When on a ketogenic diet, you are going to be in ketosis and burning through your fat stores. By incorporating exercise, you will increase you daily caloric expenditure and ramp up your fat burning. Add intermittent fasting and you'll be forced into tapping into your stored fat for longer periods of time resulting in more fat loss while simultaneously increasing your growth hormone. All this together will give you dramatic results.

The key to losing weight with ketosis and intermittent fasting is finding your maintenance level of calories and setting up a daily deficit. You will not obtain the results you want if you do not eat a calorie deficit. By incorporating a daily 16-8 intermittent fast or the occasional 24 hour fast, you can ensure you are eating a calorie deficit and derive all the benefits of fasting plus ketosis. In fact, using these two strategies together will just ensure that you are burning fat at the absolute fastest possible rate. You can eat a daily deficit while following a 16-8 fast or hit the occasional 24 hour fast to derive its fasting benefits. By following these methods, you can eat larger and more satisfying meals so the diet will be easier to follow.

So will exercising without carbohydrates hurt my results? You may have heard that you need carbohydrates in order to perform athletically. Or, that in order to have energy to workout, you must eat a sufficient amount of carbohydrates. This myth has been perpetuated for many years. Surely, cyclists and marathon athletes needs glycogen to perform proficiently. Right? Well, that's not true. In fact, studies have proven that athletic performance is not decreased in endurance and other athletes that have undergone a fat-adapted ketogenic state. So, while it may be true that when you are first undergoing ketosis, you may suffer some performance decreases and decrease in strength as your body gets adapted to ketosis, this changes the moment your body starts to rely upon your body fat as its primary energy source. After being in ketosis for a few weeks, you will have as much if not more endurance as your body is now more efficient at utilizing it's fat stores.

Will I burn up muscle mass if I workout fasted? This is another question or concern with using intermittent fasting and exercising. The concern is that by training in a fasted state, the surge in cortisol and lack of available glucose will cause your body to eat away at its protein stores (i.e. muscle) in order to fuel the brain. In order to stop this cannabalizing of the body and to prime the body for muscle growth, one should eat a good source of protein and carbohydrates at least an hour before working out. This idea that it is necessary to eat before a workout has led to all sorts of pre-workout supplementation, mostly in the form of protein powders and shakes.

The answer to the question, though, is a resounding no. You will not burn up muscle mass or hurt your progress by working out fasted. In fact, working out fasted will only speed your results and enable you to gain more muscle while burning more fat. One of the big players here that is often forgotten by the supplement companies and the spouters of bro science that proclaim you should never workout fasted is HGH. Yes, human growth hormone. One of the biggest reasons for fasting is to increase your production of HGH. Studies have shown time and time again that fasting will dramatically elevate your HGH.

Some have shown increases of up to 2000% during a 24 hour fast. As mentioned earlier, human growth hormone is responsible for such actions as promoting lean muscle mass, fat loss, and muscle growth. Since exercising also increases the production of HGH, the utilization of fasting exercises creates a synergistic environment whereas you can dramatically increase the production of this beneficial hormone. And, if you are a blossoming alpha male, exercise will increase your testosterone levels as well. Altogether, fasted exercise is a great way to optimize your results and get a super boost in your performance enhancing hormones.

Should I be concerned about losing muscle mass during a calorie deficit? This is an important question that worries most people. The fear of losing muscle mass during a weight loss period is a valid concern and especially during significant calorie deficits. However, it has been shown that as long as you are using resistance training, you will keep your lean muscle mass during calorie deficits. In fact, most bodybuilders use hardcore cutting routines for many months throughout the year to showcase their hard earned muscles without losing any lean muscle mass. The most important thing to remember here is that in order to optimize your results, you should incorporate resistance training so that you will definitely retain or increase muscle mass as your body burns up its fat reserves. The best time to incorporate this training is right before you end your fast. During this time, you will burn up more fat, have a larger HGH increase, and be able to get some protein to your muscles right after your fast in order to optimize muscle building after your workout.

When it comes to making a plan for merging your intermittent fasting and exercise plans, you are also going to need to remember that it is best to get your workout in whenever is convenient. Sure, you may optimize amino acid delivery to your muscles and thus muscle building by getting some quality protein in right after your workout but you will still derive most of the benefits if you break your fast later in the day. The most important thing in to remember is that you need to put the work in and follow the plan.

Tips for success

Strength Training is key: In order to maximize your results, you want to make sure you are doing some form of strength training. Strength training has been proven to increase fat burning and calorie expenditure more so than other forms of exercising such as jogging or walking. As well, by incorporating strength training your body will retain all of its muscle mass even during a calorie deficit. If you are new to strength training, especially, you will likely gain muscle mass while losing body fat and effectively remodel your body.

Time your workouts: In order to optimize your results, you should plan your workouts accordingly. If your main goal is fat loss, then working out in a fasted state will optimize fat burning and allow you to get more bang for your buck. However, if your goal is to stay lean while gaining muscle, you should save your workouts for periods after you have eaten and when you still have calories to consume in the day. You should wait about an hour after you have eaten to ensure that your body has metabolized the nutrients it needs, ensuring that your blood pressure is at an acceptable level and that you have lots of glycogen in your system. Once you have finished exercising it is important to consume some complex carbs along with 20 to 30 grams of protein. This will ensure that you still have glycogen left over to make it through the next day and that your body can make the most of the exercise and work to build larger muscles.

Building muscles: When strength training, experts say that you should consume anywhere between 20 and 30 grams of protein every 4 hours attaining at least one gram of protein per pound of lean body weight. As you are going to be practicing intermittent fasting at the same time, this is obviously not going to be doable. However, you should still aim to get just as much protein in your diet, just over a condensed period of time. This means you are going to want to aim for at least one gram of protein per pound of lean body weight total each day divided between one to two meals, depending upon the protocol you utilize.

If you are not going to be eating directly prior to exercising, you will want to try and time the work out so that you can eat somewhere in the neighborhood of 3 to 4 hours prior to fuel your muscles. This time frame could decrease to between 1 and 2 hours if you need to for convenience. This meal or snack should include fast acting carbs as well as blood-sugar stabilizing protein. Something like toast with peanut butter and banana is a perfect pre-workout snack. Additionally, for the best results you are going to want to try and consume 20 grams of complex carbs and 20 grams of protein within 2 hours after you have completed your workout as well.

Timing: If your type of intermittent fasting doesn't allow for the setup outlined above, you are instead going to want to aim to consume a majority of your calories in the time directly following your exercise regimen. Not only will this make it easier for your body to generate lots of lean muscle mass, it will also allow it to recover from the workout more easily. Keep in mind that if you are exercising regularly with the goal of gaining muscle you are going to want to take in approximately 500 more calories per day than you otherwise would. Alternately, if you are looking to exercise for the purpose of losing additional weight then you will need to subtract additional calories to ensure you are in a caloric deficit.

Muscle gain

So, if your main goal is to gain muscle, it can most certainly be done by utilizing a ketogenic diet and intermittent fasting. Using both of these methods together will allow you to optimize your production of HGH, increase your insulin sensitivity, boost testosterone (if male), and ultimately gain leaner muscle mass. Why should you go on a huge bulking routine and pack on a lot of fat that you will have to lose? This method will allow you to attain lean and keepable gains without the excess fat.

Train Hard and Smart. This paragraph should go without saying. If you're wanting to gain muscle mass on a keto-genic diet, then you must be training hard enough to produce a muscle building stimulus. It doesn't really matter if you'd rather train with low reps and high weights or in the more traditional body building zone of 8-10 reps. What matters is that you are getting sufficient volume and taxing yourself enough to produce the results you want. If you're wanting to maximize your muscle gains, it would also be prudent to keep cardio at a maintenance level. Too much cardio will hinder your gains and make it harder to gain weight.

Eat Sufficient Protein. In order to maximize your muscle gains, it is best to skip on the traditional ketogenic protein suggestions. Here, you will want to make sure to eat at least one gram of protein per pound of lean body mass. This will ensure that you are eating enough protein to build muscle. Don't be concerned that you will inhibit ketosis here. It is more important to ensure that you are getting enough protein. If you are working out appropriately, your body will need this amount to do what you want it to.

Eat Sufficient Calories. In order to build muscle, you will need to eat more calories than your maintenance level of calories. As discussed earlier, you should aim to start off by eating 250-500 calories over daily maintenance level to gain muscle while limiting fat gain. This is a good starting point. Start here for a couple of weeks and gauge your results. If needed, increase your calories by 250 every 1 to 2 weeks until you are gaining mass without gaining significant fat. The key here is to start low and go slow.

Add a High Carb Weekend Day. Another way to go anabolic is to add a high carb weekend day or weekend depending upon your results and preference. By increasing carbs on one day, you will replenish you glycogen stores in your muscles and be able to fuel a couple of high-intensity workouts. I would advise just doing this on one day; Friday or Saturday would be ideal. This will allow you to relax and enjoy the high carb day. You would immediately resume your ketogenic diet the next day. Ensure you also schedule a good workout the day after your carb-up. This will enable you to get a good pump and you will have tons of energy this day. Personally, I would fast until after the workout on this day but it will be up to you. When designing your carb-up day, it is good to ensure that you don't overeat so I would place a calorie limit on this day. As well, to ensure you don't pack on fat, limit your fat intake on this day. Eat sufficient protein and high carbohydrates on this day, minimizing fat intake as much as possible. If you combine your carbs and fat on this day, it will be easier to start packing on fat. Ideal foods for this day would be bagels, cereal, fruits, veggies, low fat dairy, and lean protein. Make sure you are still drinking plenty of fluids on this day as the increase carbs will dehydrate you.

Fasting Days While Building Muscle. Your fasting days will enable you to burn fat while increasing your muscle building HGH levels. Therefore, it is recommended to still utilize fasting during your quest for increased muscle mass. Ideally, a 16-8 daily intermittent fast would optimize results and be easy to stick to while getting in your daily calorie requirements. Obviously, a 24 hour fast would likely hinder weight gain so these should be used sparingly. However, a 24 hour fast does come in handy after a carb-up day or when you feel like you are packing on too much fat.

<u>*Conclusion*</u>

Thank you for making it through to the end of *Intermittent Fasting and Ketogenic Diet: How to Use Fasting to Optimize Your Ketogenic Diet: Get Leaner, Stronger, Healthier, and Better Results in Less Time,* let's hope it was informative and able to provide you with all of the tools you need to achieve your goals, whatever it is that they may be. Just because you've finished this book doesn't mean there is nothing left to learn on the topic. You can only truly learn these methods by incorporating them into your life. However, you should have everything you need to get started experimenting and truly learning this way of life.

When it comes to practicing intermittent fasting and ketogenic dieting in the long term it is important to always keep in mind that no two people are going to respond to the process in the same way. As such, you are going to want to avoid pushing your body to the breaking point, just because you want to give one of the more severe forms of intermittent fasting a try; consider working up to it instead. Always listen to what your body is trying to tell you and if you find yourself too weak to go about normal everyday tasks, stop and reassess.

With that being said, however, it is time to stop reading already and to get started planning your ketogenic diet. As well, you will need to decide what type of intermittent fasting is right for you.

It's perfectly ok to master the ketogenic diet first and then apply fasting. These two plans work perfectly together but you need to be able to execute them both to be able to reap the full benefits. Ultimately, you need to ensure you know your goals and begin planning on how and when you will reach them. As long as you dedicate yourself to the cause, you will get the results you want. By using these methods, you will find yourself leaner, stronger, more muscular, healthier, and just more badass than you ever were before.

Thank you for reading and I hope you reach your ultimate goal. If you want to learn a method of losing fat at the fastest rate possible and learn how to incorporate intermittent fasting to do so, check out my other book available on amazon

<u>Rapid Fat Loss Mastery: Lose Weight at an Incredible Rate While Retaining Muscle</u>.   This is a perfect diet to use to jump start a weight loss ketogenic diet.

Finally, if you found this book useful in anyway, a review on Amazon is always appreciated!

ABOUT THE AUTHOR

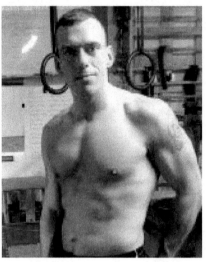

Nick Jackson is a practicing pharmacist; holding a doctorate from VCU. He also holds a precision nutrition certification in exercise nutrition, Sankyu rank in judo, and is a Snake Pit USA team member. He has an extensive background in combat sports competition; in which he has been a former Virginia judo heavyweight state champion and Tennessee State MMA Middleweight champion. He is a coach for both amateur and professional fighters at Team FAST. An avid student of nutrition, exercise, and performance disciplines, Nick is constantly pushing his limitations in his pursuit to be his best. He uses his in the trenches experience and knowledge to personally train others in martial arts, strength, conditioning, and nutrition.

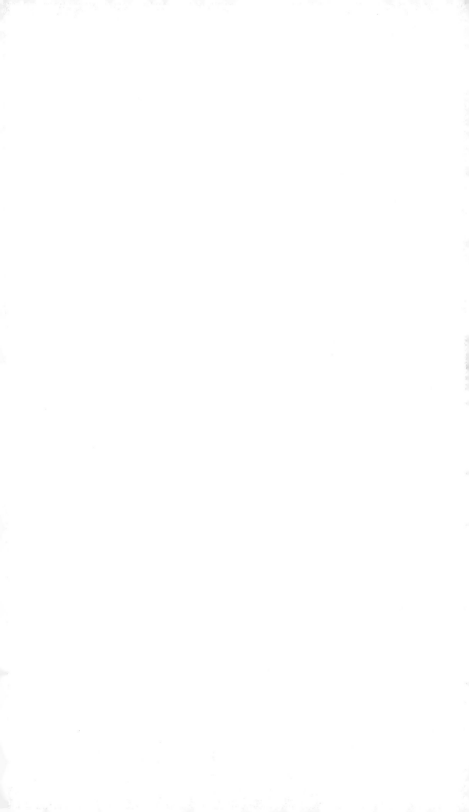

CPSIA information can be obtained
at www.ICGtesting.com
Printed in the USA
LVHW052128211218
601374LV00017B/942/P

9 781718 638587